Anatomy for th

Anatomy for the FRCA

James Bowness
Clinical Lecturer in Anaesthesia, University of Dundee
Honorary Specialty Registrar, NHS Tayside

Alasdair Taylor
Specialty Registrar, NHS Tayside

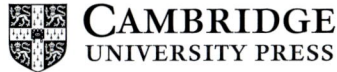

CAMBRIDGE
UNIVERSITY PRESS

University Printing House, Cambridge CB2 8BS, United Kingdom

One Liberty Plaza, 20th Floor, New York, NY 10006, USA

477 Williamstown Road, Port Melbourne, VIC 3207, Australia

314–321, 3rd Floor, Plot 3, Splendor Forum, Jasola District Centre, New Delhi – 110025, India

79 Anson Road, #06–04/06, Singapore 079906

Cambridge University Press is part of the University of Cambridge.

It furthers the University's mission by disseminating knowledge in the pursuit of education, learning, and research at the highest international levels of excellence.

www.cambridge.org
Information on this title: www.cambridge.org/9781108701884
DOI: 10.1017/9781108687805

© James Bowness and Alasdair Taylor 2019

This publication is in copyright. Subject to statutory exception and to the provisions of relevant collective licensing agreements, no reproduction of any part may take place without the written permission of Cambridge University Press.

First published 2019

Printed and bound in Great Britain by Clays Ltd, Elcograf S.p.A.

A catalogue record for this publication is available from the British Library.

Library of Congress Cataloging-in-Publication Data
Names: Bowness, James, 1983– author. | Taylor, Alasdair, 1985– author.
Title: Anatomy for the FRCA / James Bowness, Alasdair Taylor.
Description: Cambridge, United Kingdom ; New York, NY : Cambridge University Press, 2019. | Includes bibliographical references and index.
Identifiers: LCCN 2019001085 | ISBN 9781108701884 (pbk. : alk. paper)
Subjects: | MESH: Anatomy | Anesthesia–methods |
Examination Question
Classification: LCC QM32 | NLM QS 18.2 | DDC 611.0076–dc23
LC record available at https://lccn.loc.gov/2019001085

ISBN 978-1-108-70188-4 Paperback

Cambridge University Press has no responsibility for the persistence or accuracy of URLs for external or third-party internet websites referred to in this publication and does not guarantee that any content on such websites is, or will remain, accurate or appropriate.

....

Every effort has been made in preparing this book to provide accurate and up-to-date information that is in accord with accepted standards and practice at the time of publication. Although case histories are drawn from actual cases, every effort has been made to disguise the identities of the individuals involved. Nevertheless, the authors, editors, and publishers can make no warranties that the information contained herein is totally free from error, not least because clinical standards are constantly changing through research and regulation. The authors, editors, and publishers therefore disclaim all liability for direct or consequential damages resulting from the use of material contained in this book. Readers are strongly advised to pay careful attention to information provided by the manufacturer of any drugs or equipment that they plan to use.

Contents

Preface vii
Acknowledgements ix
Abbreviations x

Section 1 Question Papers

Paper 1	SAQ Exam	1
Paper 2	OSCE Exam	4
Paper 3	SOE Exams	16
Paper 4	MCQ Exam	24

Section 2 SAQs 1–12 (Answers)

SAQ 1	Base of Skull and Brain Herniation 37
SAQ 2	Brachial Plexus and Axillary Block 40
SAQ 3	Bronchial Tree and Aspiration Pneumonia 43
SAQ 4	Epidural Space and Epidural 46
SAQ 5	Femoral Triangle and Fascia Iliaca Block 48
SAQ 6	Internal Jugular Vein and Cannulation 51
SAQ 7	Intercostal Space and Chest Drain/Procedures 53
SAQ 8	Lumbar Plexus and Lumbar Plexus Block 56
SAQ 9	Oesophagus 58
SAQ 10	Pituitary Gland and Transsphenoidal Approach 60
SAQ 11	Popliteal Fossa and Block 63
SAQ 12	Trachea and Tracheostomy 66

Section 3 OSCE Stations 1–18 (Answers)

Station 1	Ankle Block 69
Station 2	Base of Skull, Foramina and Extradural Haematoma 71
Station 3	Blood Supply of the Upper Limb and Allen's Test 73
Station 4	Brachial Plexus and Supra/Infraclavicular Blocks 75
Station 5	Circle of Willis 77
Station 6	Vagus Nerve 79
Station 7	Coronary Circulation 81
Station 8	Diaphragm 84
Station 9	Dural Venous Sinuses and Cavernous Sinus Thrombosis 86

Contents

Station 10	**Inguinal Regional and Hernia** 88	SOE 1d	**Spinal Cord Blood Supply and Tracts** 118
Station 11	**Larynx** 90		
Station 12	**The Liver and Portal Venous System** 92	SOE 2a	**Trigeminal Nerve and Trigeminal Neuralgia** 121
Station 13	**Nose and Paranasal Air Sinuses** 95	SOE 2b	**Pleura and Interpleural Block** 124
Station 14	**Paravertebral Space and Block** 97	SOE 2c	**Cubital Fossa and Inadvertent Intra-Arterial Injection** 127
Station 15	**Peripheral Nerves of the Upper Limb** 99		
Station 16	**Rectus Abdominis, Sheath and Rectus Sheath Block** 101	SOE 2d	**Sacrum and Caudal Block** 130
		SOE 3a	**Scalp Block** 133
Station 17	**Ribs and Ventilation** 104	SOE 3b	**Fetal Circulation** 136
Station 18	**Vertebrae and Spinal Ligaments** 107	SOE 3c	**Blood Supply of the Lower Limb and Intraosseous Access** 139

Section 4 SOEs 1–3 (Answers)

		SOE 3d **Orbit** 142
SOE 1a	**Cervical Plexus and Carotid Endarterectomy** 109	## Section 5 MCQs 1–60 (Answers)
SOE 1b	**Anterolateral Abdominal Wall and TAP Block** 112	MCQs **T/F** 145
SOE 1c	**Brachial Plexus and Interscalene Block** 115	*References and Further Reading* 166 *Index* 167

Preface

This book has evolved from our own experience of revising for the FRCA: anatomy questions occur at all parts of the Primary or Final exams. College exam reports often cite anatomy as an area of weakness, concluding that candidates do not spend enough time preparing for this component.

The syllabus is vast and could be summarised as: anatomy [human]. Undergraduate teaching has diminished to the point of disappearing in many medical schools and, to further compound the problem, the standard of FRCA anatomy revision material can vary considerably. The mythical *greater* auricular and *posterior* tibial nerves deserve particular mention as examples of inaccurate information that have crept into the FRCA lexicon. Consequently, candidates face the laborious task of either cross-checking information from several sources or revise from a comprehensive (for which some might read 'impenetrable') non-anaesthesia anatomy text. As a result, it appears that candidates are not only unsure about anatomy, but they are also unsure where to go to learn it.

In that case, what is the best approach? Well, you could take a high-investment and low-risk strategy by learning everything. For this, you would need a more substantial and comprehensive anatomy text (we recommend *Last's Anatomy: Regional and Applied*). However, this approach is not possible for most as there is so much other material to cover. Many have previously adopted the low-investment and high-risk strategy of hoping to 'wing it'. This approach is easier during the revision stage, and it has worked for some, but you must accept the chance that a stressful, difficult and unsuccessful experience is magnified.

To respect the enormous, time-pressured challenge of the FRCA exams, we would recommend a middle road: minimise your risk whilst maximising the use of your limited time and energy investment. Targeting revision around procedures and practices that you undertake makes the anatomy relevant and will provide context, aid retention of information and assist learning for other subjects in the exam. We have therefore written this book specifically as a high-quality, reliable and accurate anatomy-specific FRCA revision aid. It covers almost all of the anatomy curriculum through a whole exam paper for each type of question in the FRCA, each focused on the anatomy and centred around clinical practice. There are 12 SAQs, 18 OSCE stations, 3 anatomy-based 4-question Final science SOEs (not just one – you lucky things!) and 60 MCQs. Candidates can focus on the particular question type most relevant to them or focus on an anatomical area by using the contents page and index. Also, remember that the anatomy content is the same regardless of how it is presented in a given type of question. For example, using the SAQ section is pretty much just as useful when studying for the Primary as for the Final, even though the Primary does not include SAQs. Also, note that human anatomy is evolving very slowly – so if you learn it well for your Primary it will still be the same for your Final! And, if you learn it well for your Final, it will stand you in good stead for your future practice/other exams (unless you take so long over your training that it has changed through evolution!).

The figures have been prepared by expert anatomy illustrators/photographers to demonstrate points in the text and aid understanding, whilst maintaining anatomical accuracy

Preface

and an appropriate level of detail. The questions have been prepared from our own knowledge as well as using several excellent publications for inspiration and reference. Whilst we have not included this information verbatim (and so have not specifically referenced them), we have cited the main sources in a 'References and Further Reading' section. We would encourage you to read these in your revision too. Particular mention should be made of the 'SLIMRAG' acronym, used throughout the book as a standard approach for answering procedural questions. This was taken from Shorthouse, Barker and Waldmann's *'SAQs for the Final FRCA'*, which the authors themselves found an excellent resource for their exam revision.

Do note that the book is a work in progress. Many of the questions have been tested by being part of our annual 'Anatomy for the FRCA' course, which is held each Spring at the School of Medicine, University of St Andrews, whilst some are new. We have striven to eradicate oversights and erroneous information, but if you feel you have spotted any (or areas of omission), we would be delighted to hear from you.

Finally, it is worth noting that the answers in this book would score highly in the FRCA. Do not be put off by the detail, embrace it instead! Solid preparation will allow you to go to London *expecting* to pass.

Study well!

Acknowledgements

Reviewers
Dr Simon Bricker (Consultant Anaesthetist, Countess of Chester Hospital, and former FRCA Examiner)
Dr Calum Grant (Consultant Anaesthetist, NHS Tayside)
Dr Ross Jones (Lecturer in Clinical and Surgical Anatomy, University of Edinburgh)

Illustrators
Mr Fraser Chisholm (photography; Prosector in the School of Medicine, University of St Andrews)
Dr Ross Jones (illustrations; Lecturer in Clinical and Surgical Anatomy, University of Edinburgh)
Dr Jeremy Mortimer (illustrations; PhD Researcher in Anatomy, University of Edinburgh)

Use of Cadaveric Material
The authors would like to thank the School of Medicine and Licensed Teacher of Anatomy at the University of St Andrews for permitting photography of cadaveric material for this book. We would also like to acknowledge the selfless contribution of those who have donated their bodies to medical science, making such educational endeavours possible.

Abbreviations

ACA	anterior cerebal artery
ARDS	acute respiratory distress syndrome
ASD	atrial septal defect
ASIS	anterior superior iliac spine
AV	atrioventricular
BP	blood pressure
CN	cranial nerve
CPP	cerebral perfusion pressure
CV	cardiovascular
CSF	cerebrospinal fluid
CVP	central venous pressure
CXR	chest X-ray
DRG	dorsal root ganglion
DVT	deep vein thrombosis
EAM	external auditory meatus
EO	external oblique
FDL	flexor digitorum longus
FHL	flexor hallucis longus
FiO_2	fraction of inspired oxygen
GA	general anaesthetic
GCS	Glasgow coma scale
GSV	great saphenous vein
IAM	internal auditory meatus
ICP	intracerebral pressure
ICS	intercostal space
IJV	internal jugular vein
ILMA	intubating laryngeal mask airway
IO	internal oblique
ITU	intensive care unit
IVC	inferior vena cava
JVP	jugular venous pulse
LCA	left coronary artery
LMA	laryngeal mask airway
MAP	mean arterial pressure
MCA	middle cerebral artery
MI	myocardial infarction
MIP	midinguinal point
MPIL	midpoint of the inguinal ligament
MS	multiple sclerosis
MTPJ	metatarsophalangeal joint
NG	nasogastric
OSA	obstructive sleep apnoea

PCA	posterior cerebral artery
PE	pulmonary embolus
PNAS	paranasal air sinuses
PSIS	posterior superior iliac spine
RCA	right coronary artery
RLN	recurrent laryngeal nerve
RV	right ventricle
SA	sinoatrial
SAD	supraglottic airway device
SVC	superior vena cava
TA	transversus abdominis
TAP	transversus abdominis plane
TCI	target-controlled infusion
TIPSS	transjugular intrahepatic portosystemic shunt
TLF	thoracolumbar fascia
VSD	ventricular septal defect

Section 1: Question Papers

Paper 1: SAQ Exam

SAQ 1

a) Where in the skull is the foramen magnum found? (1 mark)
b) Name four structures that pass through the foramen magnum (4 marks)
c) Name three types of brain herniation (3 marks)
d) Why may ocular features be a false-localising sign in brain injury causing cerebellar herniation? (2 marks)
e) Describe the pathophysiological changes of tonsillar (cerebellar) herniation (aka coning) (5 marks)
f) What hormone supplementation may be required in such patients if they are considered for brainstem death organ donation? (5 marks)

SAQ 2

a) What awake surgical procedures are permitted by the use of an axillary block? (2 marks)
b) Name the nerves targeted when performing this block and where they are found (4 marks)
c) Regarding the musculocutaneous nerve:
   i. Why may it be missed during an axillary brachial plexus block?
   ii. What does it supply?
   iii. How can a block of this nerve be supplemented? (3 marks)
d) What pattern of missed segment(s) is demonstrated in an inadequate axillary block? What areas are most likely to be spared in patients and why? What can be done to remedy this? (5 marks)
e) Describe a technique for performing an ultrasound-guided axillary brachial plexus block (6 marks)

SAQ 3

a) Describe the structure of the respiratory tree (10 marks)
b) Which segment(s) of which lung is most likely to be affected by aspiration of gastric contents (3 marks)

c) Describe the pathophysiology of aspiration pneumonitis (3 marks)
d) How do you manage aspiration in a patient with a supraglottic airway device? (4 marks)

SAQ 4

a) Describe the boundaries of the epidural space (4 marks)
b) List the contents of the epidural space (6 marks)
c) What structures does the Tuohy needle pass through when performing a midline epidural? (5 marks)
d) What are the benefits of epidural analgesia after laparotomy for malignant disease? (5 marks)

SAQ 5

a) Describe the boundaries and contents of the femoral triangle (6 marks)
b) What is a fascia iliaca block? (2 marks)
c) Describe the borders of the fascia iliaca compartment and nerves affected by the block (6 marks)
d) Describe how you would perform a fascia iliac block (6 marks)

SAQ 6

a) Describe the origin, course and termination of the internal jugular vein (IJV). Make specific reference to its relationship with the carotid artery (5 marks)
b) Describe features that distinguish the jugular venous pulse (JVP) from the carotid pulse (5 marks)
c) List five indications for cannulating the IJV (5 marks)
d) List five complications of cannulating the IJV (5 marks)

SAQ 7

a) Name the tissue layers traversed during insertion of an intercostal (chest) drain (5 marks)
b) Name and describe the muscles of the intercostal space (6 marks)
c) With the aid of a diagram, describe the structure of a spinal nerve from the T2–6 level after it has emerged from the vertebral column. State where it lies in the intercostal space (6 marks)
d) Name three procedures in anaesthesia, other than intercostal drain insertion, which make use of the intercostal space (3 marks)

SAQ 8

a) Which nerve root contributes to the lumbar plexus, in what muscle is it formed and where is the muscle found? (4 marks)
b) Name the branches of the lumbar plexus and their respective root values (6 marks)
c) Name indications and contraindications for a lumbar plexus block (5 marks)
d) What complications of regional anaesthesia are pertinent to lumbar plexus blockade? (5 marks)

SAQ 9

a) Describe the neurovascular supply of the oesophagus (9 marks)
b) List the relations of the thoracic oesophagus (4 marks)
c) What anaesthetic monitoring devices are placed in the oesophagus and what do they measure? (3 marks)
d) What features, of the distal oesophagus and surrounding structures, form the 'physiological sphincter' of the lower oesophagus to reduce reflux of gastric contents? (4 marks)

SAQ 10

a) Describe the anatomy of the pituitary gland and its relations (8 marks)
b) What is the hypothalamo-hypophyseal portal venous system? (2 marks)
c) What features of acromegaly are relevant to the conduct of general anaesthesia? (5 marks)
d) What is the transsphenoidal approach to the pituitary gland? Name the main advantages and complications (5 marks)

SAQ 11

a) What are the indications for a popliteal fossa block? (3 marks)
b) Describe the anatomy of the popliteal fossa (5 marks)
c) Describe the cutaneous innervation of the sciatic nerve below the knee (6 marks)
d) Describe a technique for performing a popliteal fossa block (6 marks)

SAQ 12

a) Briefly describe the anatomy of the trachea (6 marks)
b) List relations of the trachea in the neck (C6) and thorax (T4) (8 marks)
c) List immediate/early and late complications of a tracheostomy placed between the second and third tracheal rings (6 marks)

Section 1: Question Papers

Paper 2: OSCE Exam

Station 1

a) Name the nerves labelled A–E. Describe their area of cutaneous innervation (10 marks)
b) Identify structures F–I (4 marks)
c) Which of these nerves lie superficial to deep fascia at the level blocked? (3 marks)
d) From time of injection to onset of block, which of these nerves classically takes the longest and why? Why is it the only nerve for which a nerve stimulator would be useful? (3 marks)

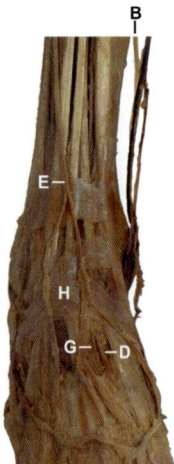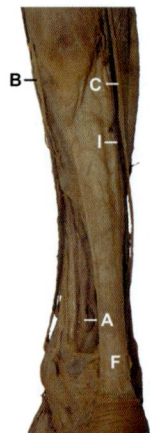

OSCE1 Dissection of dorsum of foot and posterior view of leg.

Station 2

a) From the image, name structures 1–5 and the nerves that pass through them (10 marks)
b) Name the landmarks labelled A–C and the venous sinus associated with them (3 marks)

Paper 2: OSCE Exam

c) On the image, demonstrate the boundaries of the anterior, middle and posterior cranial fossae. Describe the principal part and function of the brain associated with each (3 marks)
d) What is the name of the region indicated by D? What clinical condition is associated with trauma in this territory and why? What are the clinical features? (4 marks)

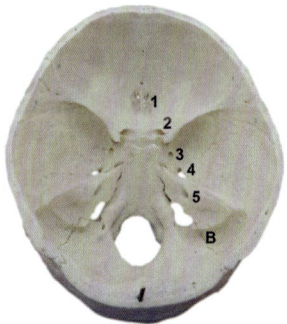 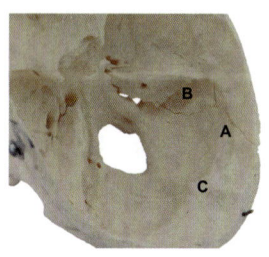 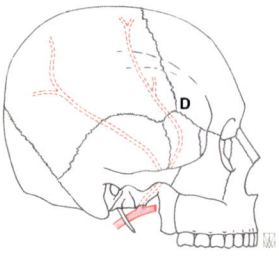

OSCE2

Station 3

a) Identify structures A–E in these cadaveric images (5 marks)
b) Name the artery running with the following nerve (3 marks):
   • Radial nerve (in the proximal arm)
   • Median nerve (in the cubital fossa)
   • Ulnar nerve (at the wrist)
c) Describe collateral arterial supply of hand (8 marks)
d) What is Allen's test? (4 marks)

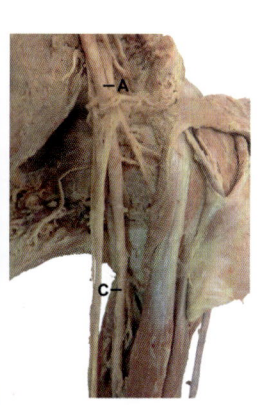 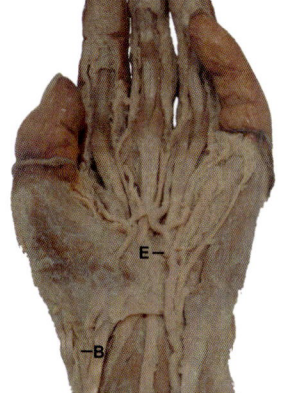 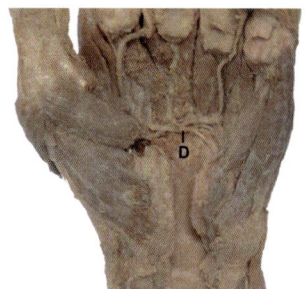

OSCE3 Dissection of anterior shoulder and palm of hand.

Station 4

a) Name structures A–E on this image of the brachial plexus (5 marks)
b) Name the nerve roots that contribute to the nerves labelled F–I (4 marks)
c) What motor response is demonstrated on stimulation of the lateral, posterior and medial cords of the brachial plexus? (3 marks)
d) Name the part(s) of the brachial plexus targeted by the following blocks (4 marks):
   - interscalene
   - supraclavicular
   - infraclavicular
   - axillary
e) What are the benefits of ultrasound-guided (over anatomical landmark or nerve stimulator) brachial plexus blocks? (4 marks)

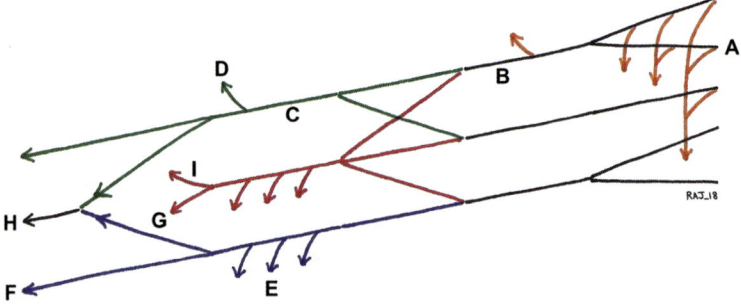

OSCE4

Station 5

a) On the image OSCE5, name structures A–E (5 marks)
b) What is the origin of A and E? (2 marks)
c) Where are the common locations of intracranial vascular aneurysms and with what frequencies do they occur? (6 marks)
d) What is the significance of the circle of Willis? (1 mark)
e) Describe the speech deficit that occurs from occlusion of the:
   i) dominant hemisphere middle cerebral artery anterior branch
   ii) dominant hemisphere middle cerebral artery posterior branch
   iii) dominant hemisphere middle cerebral artery (3 marks)
f) Which artery has been affected in a patient suffering from an occlusive stroke presenting with:
   i) motor/sensory deficit of the contralateral lower limb
   ii) contralateral homonymous hemianopia with macular sparing
   iii) motor/sensory deficit of the contralateral upper limb and face (3 marks)

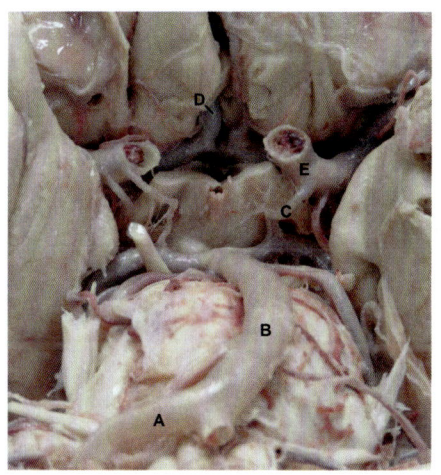 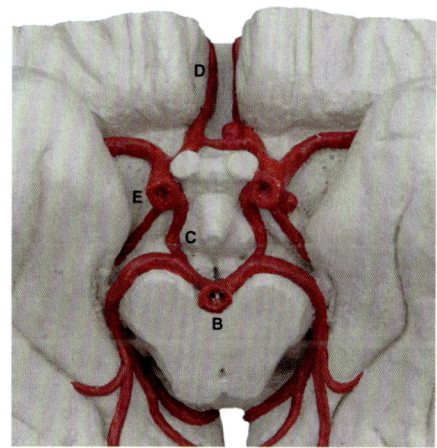

OSCE5 Cadaveric and model view of base of brain.

Station 6

a) Name the nerve labelled A on the image OSCE6 (1 mark)
b) From which nuclei does it arise? (4 marks)
c) What is the name of this foramen (B) in the base of the skull? (1 mark)
d) Which structures pass through it? (4 marks)
e) What is structure C (a branch of A)? To which vascular structure is it most closely related on the left and on the right? (4 marks)
f) What stimuli can increase the outflow of the nerve labelled A, and what effects are seen during anaesthesia? (6 marks)

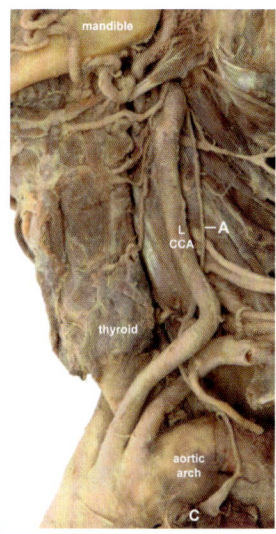 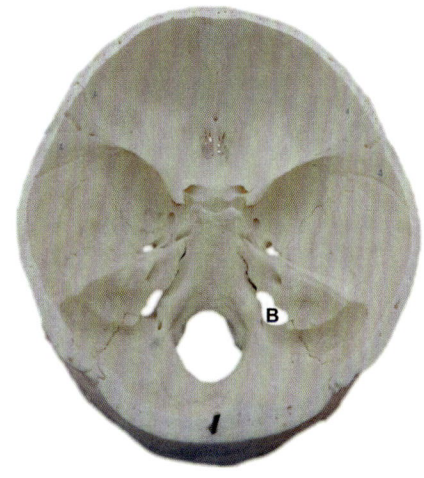

OSCE6 Dissection of left-hand side of neck (left-hand image).

Station 7

a) Name structures A–D on these images of the heart (4 marks)
b) Name structures E–H (4 marks)
c) From where do the main coronary arteries arise? (2 marks)
d) What proportion of the cardiac output is supplied to the myocardium? (1 mark)
e) What is meant by coronary arterial dominance? (1 mark)
f) Which artery supplies the AV node and where does it arise from? (2 marks)
g) Which artery supplies the SA node and where does it arise from? (2 marks)
h) What are the ECG features of right coronary artery occlusion? (2 marks)
i) Describe the difference between a type I and type II acute myocardial infarction? (2 marks)

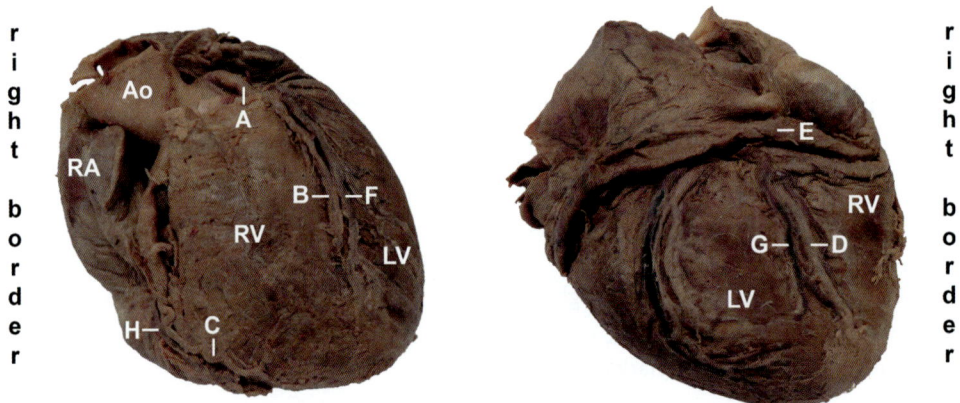

OSCE7 Anterior (sternocostal) and inferior (diaphragmatic) surfaces of the heart.

Station 8

a) On the diagram OSCE8, name structures A, B and C. State at what vertebral level they pass through the diaphragm, and name a structure they travel with at this level (9 marks)
b) What is structure D, and what is it derived from? (1 mark)
c) At which point does the left phrenic nerve pierce the diaphragm? (1 mark)
d) Describe the nerve supply of the diaphragm (3 marks)
e) What is the normal level of the diaphragm in the midclavicular line? (2 marks)
f) What are the potential causes of a raised unilateral or bilateral hemidiaphragm? (4 marks)

Paper 2: OSCE Exam

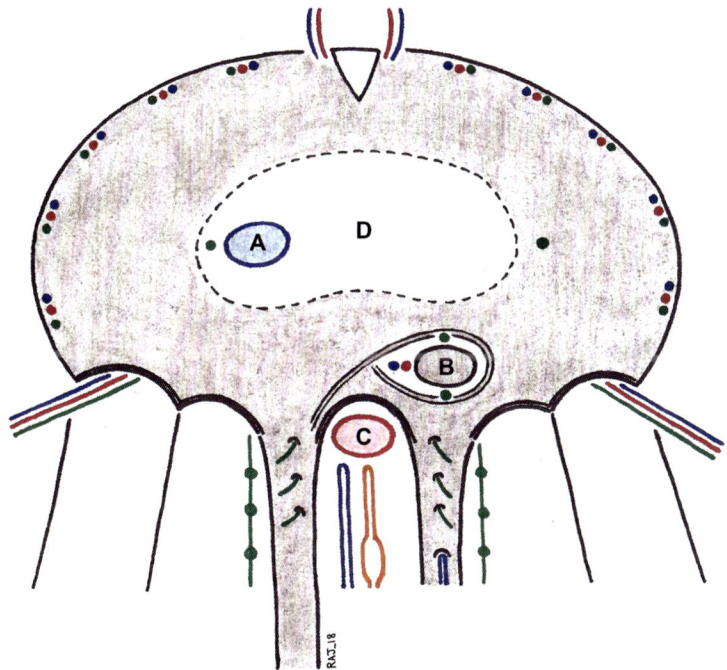

OSCE8 Illustration of the diaphragm viewed from below.

Station 9

a) Name structures A–E on the image OSCE9 (5 marks)
b) What drains to and from structure F? (5 marks)
c) What structures lie within structure F? (5 marks)
d) What are the clinical features of thrombosis of structure F? (5 marks)

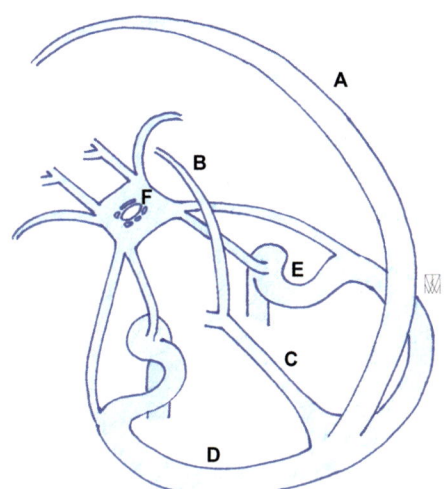

OSCE9

Station 10

a) Name structures A–F on this image (6 marks)
b) On the diagram, identify the areas supplied by the nerves numbered 1–5 (5 marks)
c) What methods of anaesthesia may be employed for inguinal hernia repair? (3 marks)
d) Describe how you would manage a patient who was having inguinal hernia repair under local anaesthesia infiltration and was beginning to experience discomfort (6 marks)

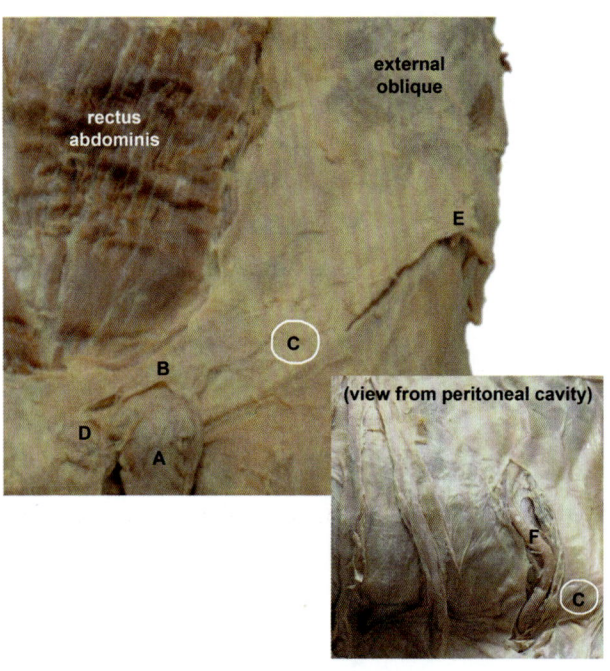
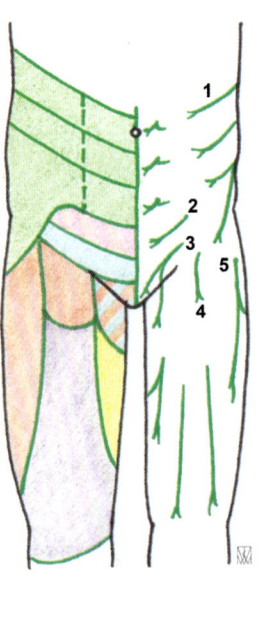

OSCE10 Dissection of the inguinal region.

Station 11

a) Name structures A–D on the diagram OSCE11 (4 marks)
b) Names structures E–I (5 marks)
c) Describe the innervation of the larynx (3 marks)
d) How might injury to the vagus nerve or its branches affect the larynx? (4 marks)
e) How can you anaesthetise the larynx for an awake fibre-optic intubation? (4 marks)

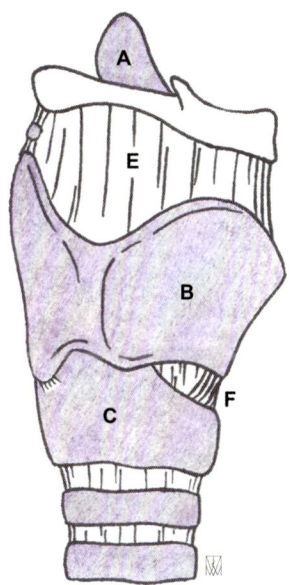
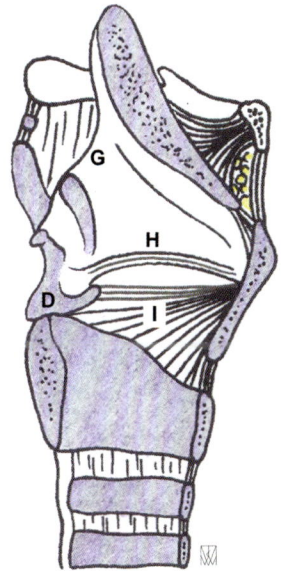

OSCE11

Station 12

a) Name structures A–E on the image OSCE12 (5 marks)
b) Describe the microscopic architecture of the liver (6 marks)
c) Name four sites of portosystemic anastomosis (4 marks)
d) Name the two vessels connected by a transjugular intrahepatic portosystemic shunt (TIPSS) procedure. How does this help to treat patients with liver cirrhosis? (5 marks)

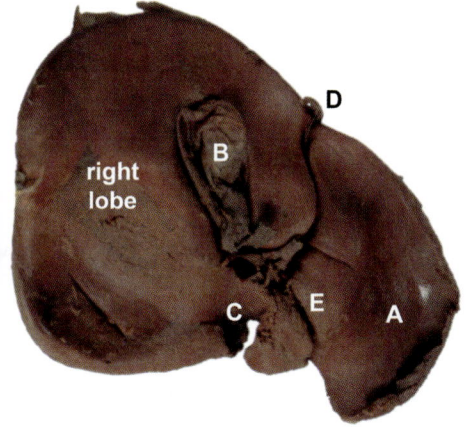

OSCE12 Inferior view of liver.

Station 13

a) Name structures 1–10 on this image of the lateral wall of the nasal cavity (10 marks)
b) Name the parent nerve from which the nerves labelled in the diagram arise (5 marks)
c) List the structures/cavities passed through, before reaching the trachea, with the fibre-optic scope when performing a nasal intubation (5 marks)

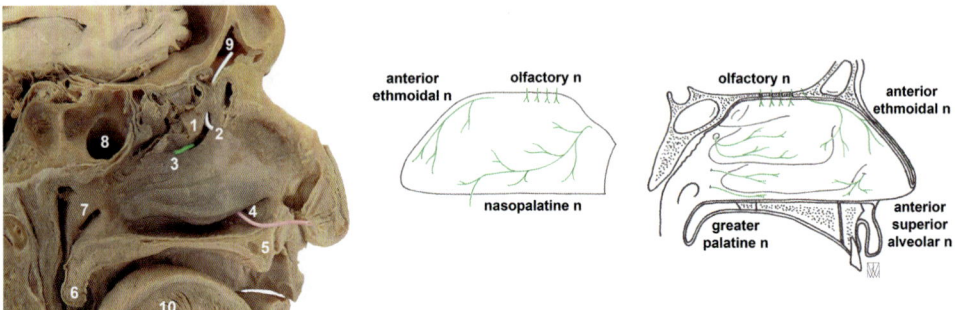

OSCE13 Cadaveric view of lateral wall of nasal cavity, mouth and pharynx, and illustrations showing innervation of septum (left)/lateral wall (right) of the nasal cavity.

Station 14

a) Name structures A–E on this diagram of the paravertebral space (5 marks)
b) Name the contents of the paravertebral space (5 marks)
c) Name four complications of paravertebral block (4 marks)
d) Describe a technique for performing a paravertebral block (6 marks)

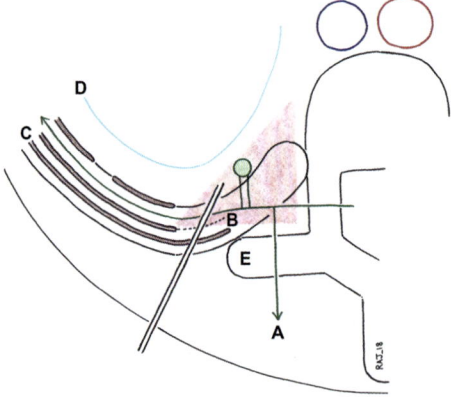

OSCE14

Paper 2: OSCE Exam

Station 15

a) Name the nerves that provide cutaneous innervation of the areas A–E in the diagram. Which one does not originate from the brachial plexus? (6 marks)
b) Name two cutaneous branches of the radial nerve in the upper limb (2 marks)
c) Name three nerves with cutaneous innervation that may be blocked in the forearm? (3 marks)
d) Name the muscle that overlies each of the following nerves in the midforearm (3 marks):
   - Median nerve
   - Ulnar nerve
   - (Superficial branch of) radial nerve
e) Describe a technique for performing an ulnar nerve block in the midforearm (6 marks)

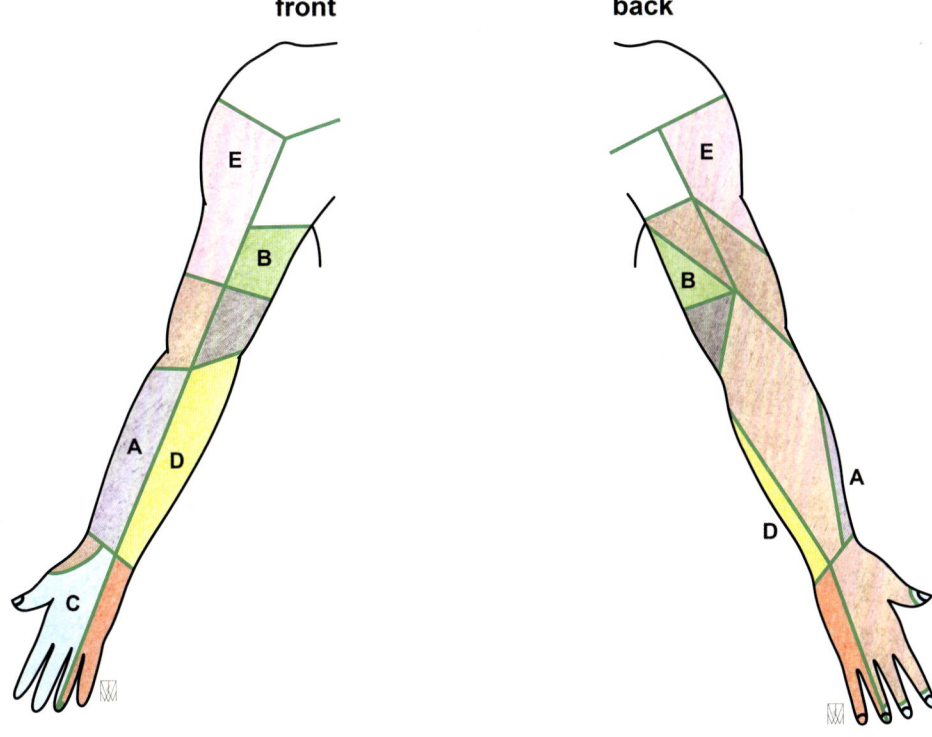

OSCE15

Station 16

a) Name the muscle in OSCE16, and describe its origin and insertion (3 marks)
b) At what level are the tendinous intersections (which give this muscle its classical appearance), and to which layer of the rectus sheath are they adherent? (2 marks)

13

c) Describe the layers and contents of the rectus sheath (6 marks)
d) Describe the regions of the following dermatomes (3 marks)
- T10
- L1
- T7
e) Describe how you would perform a rectus sheath block (6 marks)

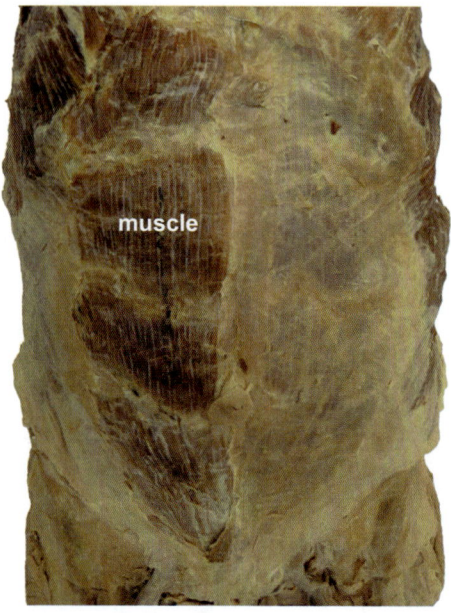

OSCE16 Dissection of the anterior abdominal wall.

Station 17

a) What is meant by the term true, false and floating ribs? (6 marks)
b) Identify the bone shown in OSCE17, and describe two ways of determining which side of the body it is from (3 marks)
c) Describe five features of the first rib that are different from/not seen on a typical rib (5 marks)
d) Describe the movements that bring about spontaneous ('negative pressure') ventilation (6 marks)

Paper 2: OSCE Exam

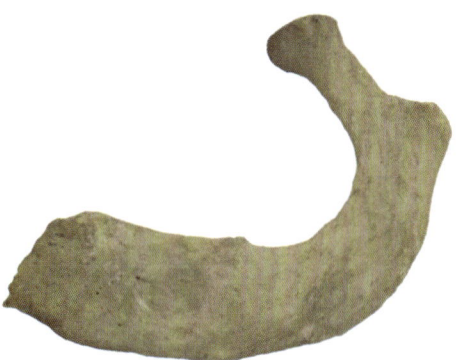

OSCE17

Station 18

a) How many vertebrae are there in the cervical, thoracic and lumbar regions of the spine? (3 marks)
b) From which regions of the spine do A, B and C originate? (3 marks)
c) What types of joint exist between vertebrae? (2 marks)
d) Do the vertebrae articulate with any other structures? (2 marks)
e) Name structures 1–4 (4 marks)
f) Which areas of the spinal column are most commonly fractured and why? (3 marks)
g) What techniques could you employ to intubate a patient with an unstable cervical spine fracture? (3 marks)

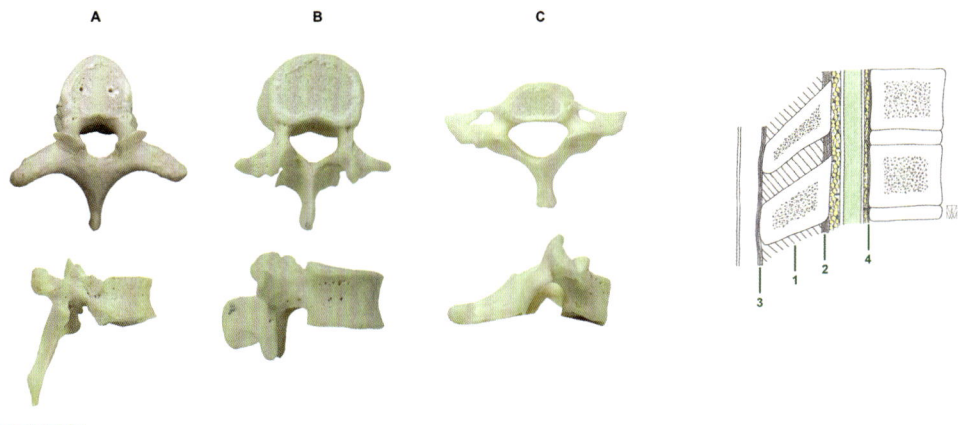

OSCE18

Section 1: Question Papers

Paper 3: SOE Exams

SOE 1

SOE 1a

a) How can anaesthesia for carotid end arterectomy be provided?
b) What nerve roots contribute to the cervical plexus, and where does this plexus lie?
c) Name the cutaneous branches of the cervical plexus (aka superficial cervical plexus) and describe their sensory distribution
d) Compare and contrast general and regional techniques of anaesthesia for carotid endarterectomy

SOE 1b

a) On the ultrasound image SOE1b, identify the muscles of the anterolateral abdominal wall (excluding rectus abdominis) and describe the orientation of their fibres
b) Describe their origin and insertion
c) In which plane does the main neurovascular bundle lie? What nerves are found here?
d) For which types of surgery may a transversus abdominis plane (TAP) block be beneficial?
e) Describe how you would perform a TAP block

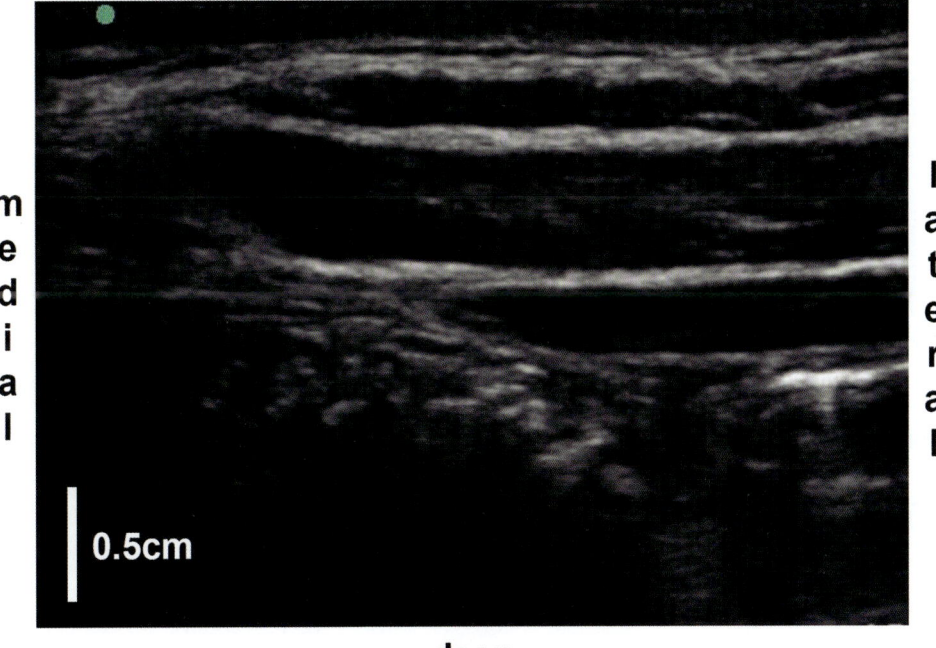

SOE1b

SOE 1c

a) On the right-hand image of SOE1c, label the dermatomes of the upper limb
b) What peripheral nerves supply the shoulder joint and skin of the shoulder region? Describe the region they supply
c) What regional anaesthesia technique may be performed to block these nerves, and which areas of the upper limb may not be blocked with this technique?
d) Name structures A–F on the ultrasound image in SOE1c of the interscalene groove
e) List the possible neurological complications of an interscalene block

Section 1: Question Papers

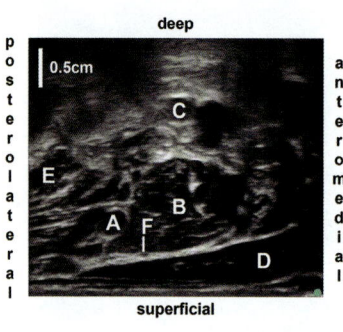
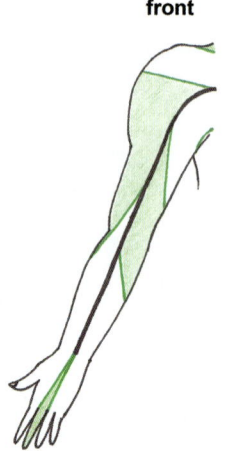
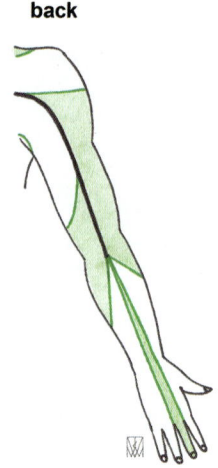

SOE1c

SOE 1d

a) Describe the blood supply to the spinal cord
b) Where are the 'watershed areas' in relation to blood supply of the spinal cord?
c) On the illustration SOE1d, label the main ascending and descending tracts in the spinal cord, and describe the signals they transmit
d) Which surgical procedures are associated with spinal cord ischaemia?
e) How can you prevent intraoperative spinal cord ischaemia?

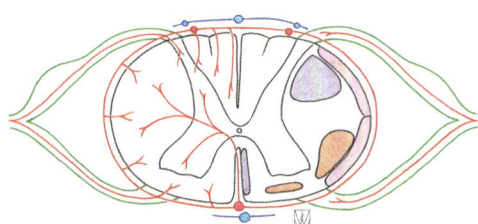

SOE1d

SOE 2

SOE 2a

a) Describe the anatomy of the trigeminal nerve (CN 5)
b) Draw a diagram to describe the sensory supply of CN 5
c) What is trigeminal neuralgia (TN)?
d) What are the risk factors and how is the diagnosis made?

e) What causes TN?
f) Describe the management of TN

SOE 2b

a) What are the pleural membranes and where are they found?
b) Describe the surface markings of the pleura with reference to the photograph of the thoracic skeleton
c) What are the costodiaphragmatic and costomediastinal recesses and where are they found?
d) Describe the innervation of the pleura
e) What are the indications for an interpleural block?
f) Outline how to perform an interpleural block

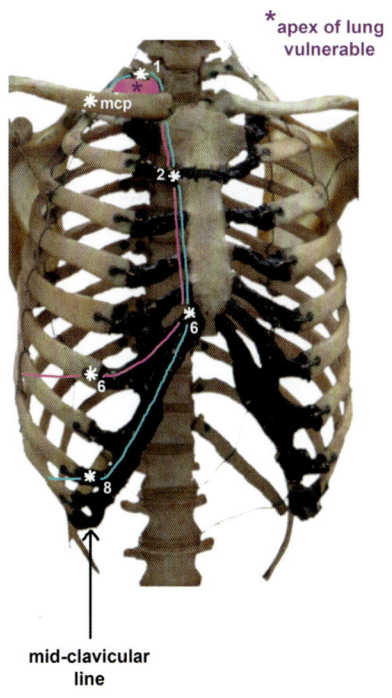
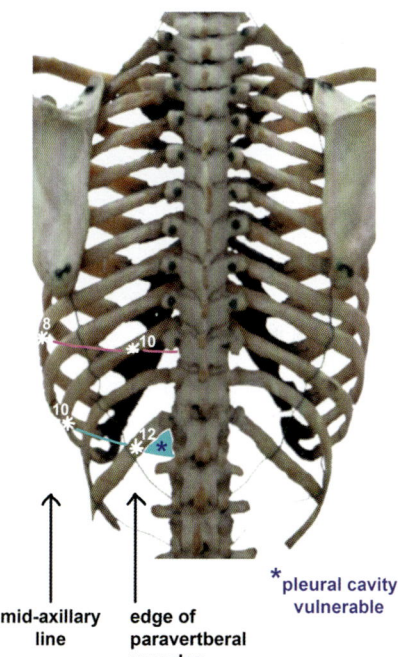

SOE2b

SOE 2c

a) Describe the boundaries of the cubital fossa with reference to the cadaveric image SOE2c
b) What are the contents of the cubital fossa?
c) Name the superficial veins associated with the cubital fossa, the areas they drain and where they drain to
d) What are the features of inadvertent intra-arterial injection here?

e) Why is intra-arterial injection of thiopentone problematic?
f) How would you manage a patient who has just received inadvertent intra-arterial injection of thiopentone?

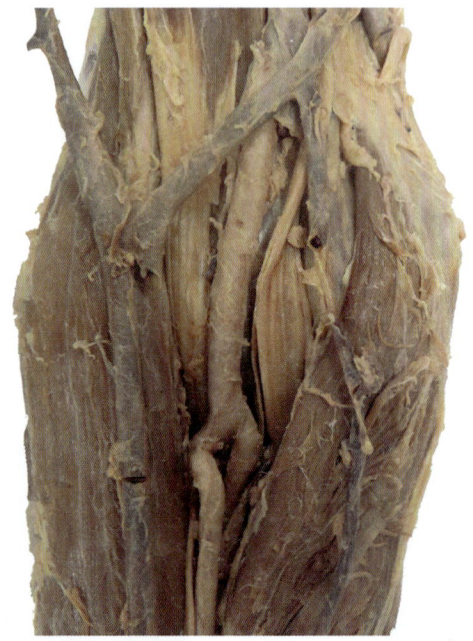

SOE2c Dissection of the cubital fossa.

SOE 2d

a) A six-month-old, otherwise well, boy is to undergo general anaesthesia for an inguinal hernia repair. What analgesic options would you consider?
b) For what type of surgery may a caudal block provide adequate analgesia?
c) Describe the anatomy of the sacrum
d) What are the anatomical considerations with regard to paediatric neuroaxial blockade?
e) How can you identify the sacral hiatus?
f) What dose of 0.25% levo-bupivacaine would you use for this surgery?
g) What are the contraindications and complications of a caudal block?

SOE 3

SOE 3a

a) On the image SOE3a, name the (seven pairs of) nerves targeted in a scalp block. Describe the region they supply.
b) Which of these nerves are derived from cranial nerves (and from which one)?
c) What are the indications for a scalp block?
d) What landmarks are used to block each of these nerves as part of a scalp block?

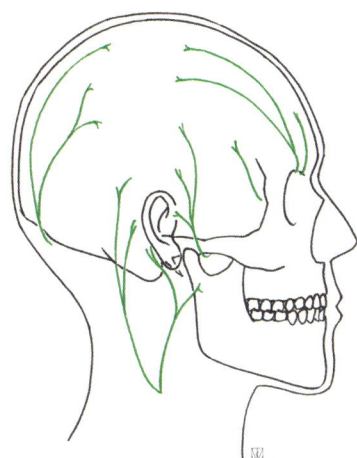

SOE3a

SOE 3b

a) Use the diagram SOE3b to describe the fetal circulation, starting at the umbilical vein
b) Label the diagram with approximate oxygen saturation of blood at the following points:
   - Umbilical vein
   - IVC
   - Ascending aorta
   - Ductus arteriosus
   - Descending aorta
c) What are the physiological changes that occur at birth?
d) Describe the development and structure of the foramen ovale
e) What is meant by a paradoxical embolus?

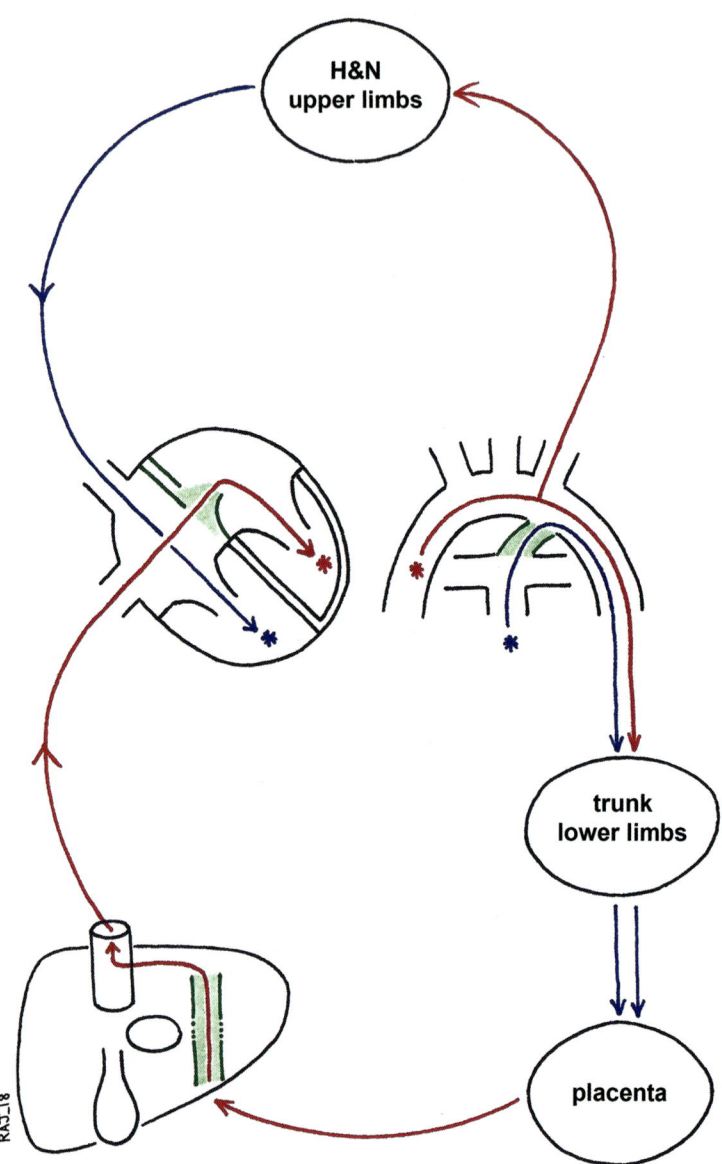

SOE3b

SOE 3c

a) Describe the arterial supply of the lower limb
b) Describe the course of the great/long saphenous vein
c) Name the principal superficial vein on the posterior surface of the leg
d) With which nerves do these two veins run in the leg?

e) Name two sites for intraosseous vascular access in the lower limb
f) Name the indications and contraindications to intraosseous access

SOE 3d

a) Describe the bony structure of the orbit
b) On this image of the orbit, identify features A–E
c) Which areas do A and B run between, and what structures do they transmit?
d) What is the nerve supply to the eye?
e) What blocks are used to provide anaesthesia in surgery on the eye?

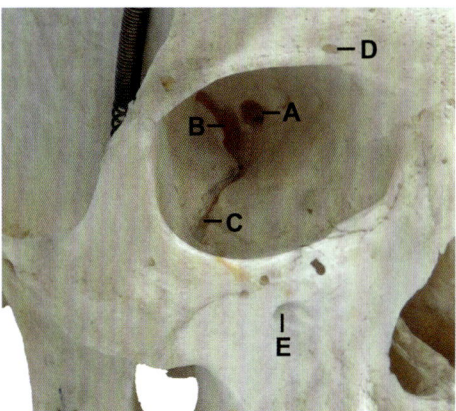

SOE3d

Section 1: Question Papers

Paper 4

MCQ Exam
True or False

1. **The anterior triangle of the neck:**
   - Is bounded posteriorly by the anterior border of sternocleidomastoid
   - Contains the carotid sheath
   - Contains the external jugular vein
   - Is overlain by skin supplied by the transverse cervical nerve(s)
   - Is bounded superiorly by the lower border of the mandible

2. **Regarding the anterolateral abdominal wall:**
   - The lumbar triangle (of Petit) is bounded by the posterior border of the external oblique muscle, the anterior border of the latissimus dorsi muscle and the iliac crest
   - The floor of the lumbar triangle (of Petit) is formed by the transversus abdominis muscle
   - During a landmark technique TAP block, two 'pops' are felt as the needle passes through the thoracolumbar fascia and external oblique layer
   - A subcostal TAP block can be used for surgery extending above the umbilicus
   - The external oblique, internal oblique and transversus abdominis muscles all have the same innervation, which is solely from the thoracoabdominal (T7–11) and subcostal (T12) nerves

3. **At the ankle:**
   - All of the deep nerves supplying the foot are branches of the sciatic nerve
   - The deep peroneal nerve enters the dorsum of the foot between the tendons of extensor hallucis longus and extensor digitorum longus
   - The deep peroneal nerve is a hyperechoic structure on ultrasound
   - The superficial peroneal nerve emerges between extensor digitorum longus and peroneus brevis
   - The sural nerve lies anterior to the medial malleolus

4. **Regarding the larynx and trachea:**
   - In the adult, the narrowest part of the upper respiratory tract is at the level of the cricoid cartilage
   - In the child, the narrowest part of the upper respiratory tract is at the level of the (open) vocal cords
   - The position of the carina moves with respiration
   - The trachea is in contact with the left vagus nerve in the thorax
   - The trachea is in contact with the thoracic duct posteriorly

5. **The following is true of the ribs:**
   - The sympathetic trunk is an anterior relation of the neck of the first rib
   - Typical ribs have a head with two articular facets, for articulation with their own vertebra and the one below
   - Typical ribs have a tubercle with a smooth articular facet, which forms a synovial joint with the transverse process of the corresponding vertebra
   - Typical ribs have a tubercle with a rough non-articular facet, for attachment of the lateral costotransverse ligament
   - The costal cartilages of ribs 2–10 form primary cartilaginous joints with the sternum or rib/costal cartilage above

6. **Regarding autonomic dysreflexia:**
   - Excess sympathetic discharge occurs in response to stimuli below level of spinal cord lesion
   - Features are more pronounced with higher lesions and a stronger reaction is observed if a more proximal dermatome is stimulated
   - Patients develop tachycardia/arrhythmias, with severe hypotension and headache
   - Below the level of the spinal cord lesion, patients exhibit sweating, pallor and muscle contraction/spasticity
   - Central neuroaxial blockade can be used to prevent and manage autonomic dysreflexia

7. **The following are true of the internal auditory meatus/auditory canal:**
   - It transmits the vestibulocochlear nerve and the facial nerve
   - It is directed laterally in the petrous bone
   - It connects the middle cranial fossa to the inner ear
   - It contains only the motor component of CN 7
   - The vestibular ganglion lies within the internal auditory meatus

8. **Regarding the rectus abdominis:**
   - The rectus abdominis muscle lies superficial to the external oblique aponeurosis
   - The superior epigastric artery is a branch of the internal thoracic artery
   - The arcuate line of the rectus sheath lies approximately halfway between the pubic symphysis and umbilicus
   - Motor supply of the rectus abdominis is partly by the iliohypogastric nerve
   - Perforation of the inferior epigastric artery is a common complication of rectus sheath block

9. **The following is true of the lower limb vasculature:**
   - The femoral artery lies in the adductor (subsartorial/Hunter's) canal
   - The inferior epigastric artery is a branch of the femoral artery
   - The femoral vein lies medial to the femoral artery initially, but lies posteriorly to it at the apex of the femoral triangle
   - The popliteal vein is the deepest structure in the popliteal fossa
   - The peroneal artery provides little or no arterial supply to the foot

10. **Regarding the scalp block:**
    - The infraorbital nerve is targeted
    - The transverse cervical nerves are targeted
    - The third occipital nerve is targeted
    - A scalp block can be the sole technique used for awake craniotomy, without sedation or general anaesthesia, as the brain itself is not sensitive to painful stimuli
    - Intra-arterial injection into the superficial temporal artery is possible when targeting the auriculotemporal nerve

11. **Regarding the lungs and pleura:**
    - The pulmonary ligament consists of pleura
    - The visceral pleura has no sensory innervation
    - At the midpoint between full inspiration and expiration, the inferior border of the lung lies at the level of the sixth rib in the midclavicular line
    - The horizontal fissure of the right lung lies at the level of the fourth costal cartilage and runs horizontally backwards to meet the oblique fissure in the midaxillary line
    - The blunt posterior border of the lung lies in the paravertebral gutter, either side of the midline

12. **Regarding Brown–Séquard syndrome:**
    - It typically results after complete transection of the spinal cord
    - It results in an ipsilateral upper motor neurone lesion (spastic paralysis) below the level of the injury
    - It results in an ipsilateral lower motor neurone lesion (flaccid paralysis) below the level of the injury
    - It results in ipsilateral loss of vibration sensation and proprioception (dorsal column) below the level of the injury
    - It results in contralateral loss of pain and temperature sensation (spinothalamic tract) below the level of the injury

13. **The following bones contribute to the pterion:**
    - Sphenoid (greater wing)
    - Frontal
    - Temporal (squamous part)
    - Parietal
    - Occipital

14. **Regarding the bronchial circulation:**
    - The bronchial arteries supply the lung parenchyma with oxygenated blood
    - The bronchial arteries arise from the corresponding pulmonary artery
    - There are two bronchial arteries supplying the right lung
    - The bronchial veins return deoxygenated blood directly to the inferior vena cava
    - The bronchial and pulmonary circulations allow mixing of oxygenated and deoxygenated blood

15. **Regarding the blood supply of the upper limb:**
    - The axillary artery is a continuation of the subclavian artery at the lateral border of scalenus anterior
    - The cords of the brachial plexus are named according to their relationship to the second part of the axillary artery
    - The axillary artery gives rise to medial and lateral circumflex humeral arteries
    - The ulnar artery gives rise to the common interosseous artery
    - The superficial (palmar) branch of the radial artery travels into the hand deep to the flexor retinaculum

16. **The following is true regarding relations of the orbit:**
    - The anterior cranial fossa is a superior relation of the orbit
    - The ethmoid air sinuses are a medial relation of the orbit
    - The sphenoid air sinus is a posterior relation of the orbit
    - The maxillary air sinus is a medial relation of the orbit
    - The infratemporal fossa and middle cranial fossa are posterolateral relations of the orbit

17. **Which of the following are boundaries of the paravertebral space?**
    - The superior costotransverse ligament is a superior boundary
    - The visceral pleura of the thorax is an anterolateral boundary
    - The psoas muscle is an anterolateral boundary at the lumbar level
    - The endothoracic fascia is a medial boundary
    - The vertebral body is a medial boundary

18. **Regarding central cord syndrome:**
    - It is commonly due to a crush injury (without transection) of the spinal cord
    - Hyperextension of the cervical spine is a common feature
    - The upper limbs are affected more than the lower limbs
    - The cervical fibres of the spinothalamic tract are more superficial than the sacral fibres
    - The anterior horn of grey matter is not affected

19. **Regarding sutures of the cranium:**
    - They are secondary cartilaginous joints
    - They fuse at around 20–40 years of age
    - The lambda represents the closed/ossified posterior fontanelle
    - The anterior fontanelle closes/ossifies after the posterior fontanelle
    - An extradural haematoma crosses lines of sutural intersection

20. **The following is true in relation to the right lung root:**
    - The right upper lobe bronchus and accompanying artery are found above the main bronchus
    - The pulmonary arteries lie anterior to their respective bronchi
    - Four pulmonary veins drain the lung
    - Branches of the phrenic nerve supply the lung parenchyma
    - Pulmonary lymphatics drain the lung via this route

21. **Regarding the brachial plexus:**
    - It comprises five roots, three trunks, five divisions and three cords
    - The branching pattern of the brachial plexus often varies between the right and left sides in the same individual
    - The sheath surrounding the brachial plexus is at its smallest volume in the supraclavicular fossa
    - The roots lie anterior to the anterior scalene muscle
    - It provides motor innervation to the serratus anterior muscle

22. **The following bones contribute to the orbital margin/rim:**
    - Frontal
    - Zygomatic
    - Maxilla
    - Nasal
    - Ethmoid

23. **Concerning the oesophageal sphincters:**
    - Atropine reduces lower oesophageal sphincter pressure
    - The lower oesophageal sphincter is in a state of tonic contraction
    - The upper oesophagus consists of skeletal muscle, but is not under voluntary control
    - Upper oesophageal sphincter tone is reduced by all intravenous anaesthetic induction agents
    - Upper oesophageal sphincter tone is reduced by both non-depolarising and depolarising neuromuscular blocking drugs

24. **Regarding anterior spinal artery syndrome:**
    - Proprioception is preserved below the level of the lesion
    - Voluntary motor function is lost below the level of the lesion
    - An upper motor neurone lesion (spastic paralysis) will develop below the level of the lesion
    - Pain and temperature sensation is preserved below the level of the lesion
    - The lateral spinothalamic tract is typically affected

25. **The carotid sheath:**
    - Contains the external carotid artery
    - Contains the internal jugular vein
    - Contains the recurrent laryngeal nerve
    - Contains the ansa cervicalis within its anterior wall
    - Lies anterior to the phrenic nerve

26. **Regarding the coronary circulation:**
    - There are no anastomoses between the regions of arterial supply in the heart
    - 80–90% of coronary venous circulation is returned to the right atrium via the coronary sinus
    - Blood supply to the right ventricle ceases during systole
    - The myocardium typically extracts approximately 50% of oxygen from arterial blood

- The right ventricle is mainly supplied by the right coronary artery, originating from the proximal pulmonary trunk

27. **Regarding the brachial plexus:**
    - The divisions lie in the infraclavicular fossa
    - The trunks lie anterior to the subclavian artery
    - The three cords are described in relation to the subclavian artery
    - Pectoralis major lies anterior to the cords
    - The supraclavicular nerve typically branches from the upper trunk

28. **CN 3 (the oculomotor nerve) supplies the following muscles of the orbit/eye:**
    - Lateral rectus
    - Superior oblique
    - Levator palpebrae superioris
    - Medial rectus
    - Dilator muscle of the iris

29. **Regarding oesophageal pathology:**
    - Boerhaave's syndrome refers to oesophageal rupture secondary to iatrogenic injury
    - Nasogastric tube placement is contraindicated in the presence of oesophageal varices
    - Achalasia refers to failure of the lower oesophageal sphincter to relax
    - Adenocarcinoma of the oesophagus occurs mainly in the distal third
    - Approximately 80% of oesophageal cancer occurs in men

30. **The following is true with regard to adult and paediatric neuroaxial blockade:**
    - The spinal cord ends at L1/2 in adults, but lower in children
    - The dura ends at S2 in adults, but higher in children
    - The subarachnoid space extends into the sacral canal
    - The male sacrum displays a greater curvature than the female sacrum
    - The sacrum articulates with four bones

31. **The following is true of the muscular branches of the cervical plexus (aka deep cervical plexus):**
    - The phrenic nerve (C3/4/5) is not a branch of the cervical plexus
    - The parietal pleura receives sensory innervation from a muscular branch of the cervical plexus
    - The ansa cervicalis (C1–3) forms part of this plexus
    - Branches from C2/3 and C3/4 transmit proprioceptive sensation from sternocleidomastoid and trapezius
    - The cervical plexus does not innervate any structures inside the cranial cavity

32. **Regarding the diaphragm:**
    - The central part is derived from the pleuroperitoneal membranes
    - The central tendon is derived from the septum transversum
    - It arises in part from the lateral arcuate ligament

- The sympathetic chain enters the abdomen behind the medial arcuate ligament
- The median arcuate ligament forms the aortic hiatus

33. **Regarding the axillary brachial plexus block:**
    - It reliably blocks the intercostobrachial nerve
    - Motor innervation to biceps brachii is via the musculocutaneous nerve
    - The axillary artery typically lies posterior to the conjoint tendon of teres major and latissimus dorsi
    - The musculocutaneous nerve appears as a hypoechoic structure, due to the lack of connective tissue
    - The axillary nerve is normally blocked

34. **Regarding the orbit:**
    - The inferior orbital fissure transmits the zygomatic branch of the maxillary nerve
    - The inferior orbital fissure transmits the inferior division of CN 3
    - The supraorbital nerve passes through the supraorbital notch to supply the frontal belly of the occipitofrontalis
    - The infraorbital foramen lies in the zygomatic bone
    - The infraorbital nerve supplies skin from the lower eyelid to the chin

35. **The oesophagus:**
    - Is approximately 25 cm long in the adult
    - Has no outer serosal covering
    - Inclines to the right as it descends in the inferior part of the thorax
    - Lymph travels relatively large distances in the wall of the oesophagus before reaching the regional lymph nodes
    - Drains largely to the systemic venous circulation

36. **The radial nerve:**
    - Is derived from roots C5–T1
    - Provides the principal motor supply to biceps brachii
    - Courses around the surgical neck of the humerus
    - Gives motor innervation to the medial and lateral heads of triceps brachii
    - Can be reliably blocked using ultrasound at the midforearm level

37. **Regarding CN 5 (the trigeminal nerve):**
    - It is the largest calibre cranial nerve
    - The ophthalmic division provides motor supply to the levator palpebrae superioris muscle
    - The mandibular division supplies the sensation of taste to the anterior two-thirds of the tongue
    - Loss of the corneal reflex is consistent with a CN 5 lesion
    - The mandibular division provides sensory supply to the temporomandibular joint

38. **Regarding the fetal circulation:**
    - All of the blood in the umbilical vein enters the right atrium
    - The three fetal shunts normally close immediately after birth

- Blood perfusing the brain of the fetus has the same PaO2 as that of the descending aorta
- The foramen ovale remains patent in 25%
- Blood travelling to the fetus via the umbilical vein is fully saturated with oxygen

39. **Regarding the cubital fossa:**
    - The brachial artery provides the entire blood supply to the hand
    - The brachial artery usually divides into the radial and ulnar arteries at the apex of the cubital fossa
    - The posterior interosseous nerve arises from the median nerve in the cubital fossa
    - Sensory innervation to the medial border of the hand and fifth finger is provided by the median nerve
    - The biceps tendon lies medial to the brachial artery

40. **Regarding the nose and paranasal air sinuses:**
    - The maxillary air sinus is the largest sinus
    - The nasal septum is partly formed from hyaline cartilage
    - The blood supply of the septal cartilage is from overlying perichondrium
    - CN 1 (olfactory nerve) innervates only the neuroepithelium of the upper nasal cavity (including its roof and upper parts of the medial/lateral walls)
    - The nasolacrimal duct drains the lacrimal sac to the inferior meatus of the nasal cavity

41. **The following is true of the fetal circulation:**
    - 50% of the cardiac output passes through the pulmonary capillaries
    - Prostaglandin analogues can be used to influence closure of the ductus arteriosus
    - The Eustachian valve directs oxygenated blood from the SVC into the pulmonary artery
    - The ligamentum teres of the abdomen and the ligamentum venosum are continuous
    - The umbilical arteries obliterate and become the medial umbilical ligament

42. **The epidural space:**
    - Contains the sympathetic chains
    - Is continuous with the sacral canal
    - Has no lymphatic drainage
    - Lies posterior to the posterior longitudinal ligament
    - Contains no free fluid in health

43. **Regarding the larynx:**
    - The epiglottis is formed from hyaline cartilage
    - The superior laryngeal artery pierces the thyrohyoid membrane with the internal branch of the superior laryngeal nerve
    - The cricothyroid muscle elongates the vocal cords
    - The vocalis muscle tenses the vocal cords
    - The cricoarytenoid joint is a synovial joint

44. **The lumbar plexus:**
    - Receives a contribution from the L5 nerve root in half of the population
    - Can be seen as a hyperechoic area within the posterior third of the psoas muscle
    - Is reliably blocked by the '3 in 1' block
    - Induces hamstring contraction (knee flexion) as the desired end point/motor response when using a peripheral nerve stimulator to guide correct needle placement
    - Gives only mixed nerves (with motor and sensory fibres)

45. **Regarding a sciatic nerve block in the popliteal fossa:**
    - Stimulation of the tibial nerve produces plantar flexion of the ankle/toes and inversion of the foot
    - Stimulation of the common peroneal (fibular) nerve produces dorsiflexion of the ankle/toes, eversion of the foot
    - Sciatic nerve block proximally in the thigh will provide anaesthesia and immobility to the knee
    - The sciatic nerve provides all of the cutaneous innervation to the foot
    - The posterior cutaneous nerve of the thigh, which provides cutaneous innervation over the posterior thigh and popliteal fossa, is a branch of the sciatic nerve

46. **Muscles whose motor supply is from CN 5 (the trigeminal nerve) include:**
    - Temporalis
    - Buccinator
    - Medial and lateral pterygoids
    - Levator palati
    - Posterior belly of digastric muscle

47. **The following is true of the heart:**
    - The pericardium is composed of three layers
    - In a healthy patient, around 50% of the heart lies to the right of the midline
    - The primary chamber comprising the base (posterior surface) of the heart receives four pulmonary veins
    - Only 50% of the coronary circulation drains into the coronary sinus
    - The coronary sinus contains no valves, thus cardioplegia solution can be injected retrogradely through it to arrest the myocardium

48. **Regarding the structures of the proximal anterior thigh:**
    - The femoral nerve is found at the midinguinal point as it enters the thigh, immediately below the inguinal ligament
    - The femoral artery is found at the midinguinal point as it enters the thigh, immediately below the inguinal ligament
    - The femoral nerve does not supply any structures in the abdominopelvic cavity
    - The superficial (anterior) group of femoral nerve branches are purely sensory
    - The deep (posterior) group of femoral nerve branches are purely motor

49. **The internal jugular vein:**
    - Exits the middle cranial fossa through the jugular foramen
    - The superior, middle and inferior thyroid veins all drain to the IJV

- Lies within the carotid sheath
- Lies deep to the investing fascia of the neck
- Continues as the subclavian vein behind the medial end of the clavicle

50. **Regarding neurocardiology:**
    - Parasympathetic supply to the heart is only partly from CN 10 (vagus nerve)
    - The sympathetic outflow to the heart is from spinal levels T1–T4
    - The autonomic plexus supplying the heart is divided into two parts
    - The sinoatrial node lies in the wall of the right atrium, just below the SVC
    - The atrioventricular node lies in the interventricular septum

51. **The following are cutaneous branches of the femoral nerve:**
    - Medial cutaneous nerve of the thigh
    - Intermediate cutaneous nerve of the thigh
    - Lateral cutaneous nerve of the thigh
    - Posterior cutaneous nerve of the thigh
    - Saphenous nerve

52. **Regarding the dura and venous circulation of the cranium:**
    - The tentorium cerebelli lies between the occipital lobes and the cerebellum
    - The tentorium cerebelli contains no dural venous sinus in its lateral/posterior (fixed) margin
    - The superior petrosal sinus drains the cavernous sinus to the transverse sinus
    - Arachnoid villi are protrusions of the arachnoid mater into the subarachnoid space to allow filtration of blood for the production of CSF
    - Venous blood from deep regions of the brain drain via the great cerebral vein (of Galen) to the straight sinus

53. **Regarding the blood supply of the liver and bowel:**
    - The common hepatic artery only supplies the liver
    - The superior mesenteric vein drains the foregut
    - The midgut extends from the midpoint of the second part of the duodenum to the junction of the proximal two-thirds and distal third of the transverse colon
    - The hindgut extends from the distal third of the transverse colon to the upper half of the anal canal
    - The portal vein drains deoxygenated blood from the liver to the inferior vena cava

54. **Regarding the popliteal fossa:**
    - The short saphenous vein is found in the popliteal fossa
    - The sciatic nerve rarely divides proximal to the apex of the popliteal fossa
    - The sural nerve receives contributions from both tibial and common peroneal (fibular) nerves
    - The sural nerve runs with the short saphenous vein
    - Popliteus muscle is supplied by the common peroneal (fibular) nerve

Section 1: Question Papers

55. **Regarding CN 10 (the vagus nerve):**
    - The left vagus nerve passes over the arch of the aorta
    - The right recurrent laryngeal nerve enters the thorax before passing under the subclavian artery
    - The left vagus nerve is a direct relation of the trachea in the thorax
    - The right vagus nerve contributes predominantly to the anterior vagal trunk
    - The vagal trunks pass through the diaphragm with the oesophagus at the level of T10

56. **The following is true of spinal nerves:**
    - There are seven pairs of cervical spinal nerves (corresponding to the seven cervical vertebrae)
    - The dorsal root ganglion contains cell bodies of sensory nerves, but no synapses
    - The anterior root of every spinal nerve contains both motor and autonomic fibres
    - A white ramus communicans is associated with every spinal nerve
    - Both the anterior and posterior divisions (rami) of spinal nerves contribute to the main cervical, brachial, lumbar and sacral plexuses

57. **Regarding innervation of the upper limb:**
    - The ulnar nerve provides motor supply to adductor pollicis
    - The deep branch of the radial nerve provides sensory supply to the dorsum of the hand
    - The ulnar nerve provides sensation to the medial aspect of the forearm, proximal to the wrist
    - Radial nerve palsy, due to fracture of the shaft of the humerus, leads to an inability to extend the elbow joint
    - The musculocutaneous nerve provides no sensory innervation to the hand

58. **CN 12 (the hypoglossal nerve):**
    - Is a paired nerve comprising both spinal and cranial roots
    - Exits the skull through the hypoglossal canal in the temporal bone
    - A unilateral lesion of this nerve will cause the tongue to deviate to the unaffected side
    - Carries motor and sensory fibres
    - Courses through the carotid sheath

59. **Regarding the thoracic spinal nerves:**
    - The anterior division (ramus) lies anterior to the internal thoracic artery in the upper six intercostal spaces
    - The intercostal nerve is the most inferior structure of the main intercostal neurovascular bundle
    - They provide a recurrent nerve to the vertebral canal, which provides sensory supply to the dura and arachnoid
    - The first intercostal nerve (T1) provides nerve fibres for the brachial plexus but not the first intercostal space
    - The second intercostal nerve (T2) provides supply to the axilla

60. **Regarding innervation of the upper limb:**
    - Sensory innervation to the thumb is provided by the median and radial nerves
    - The ulnar nerve supplies skin proximal to the wrist
    - The radial nerve supplies all three heads of triceps brachii
    - The radial nerve supplies the adductor pollicis muscle
    - The median nerve provides the sole motor supply to flexor digitorum profundus

Section 2 SAQs 1–12 (Answers)

SAQ 1

Base of Skull and Brain Herniation

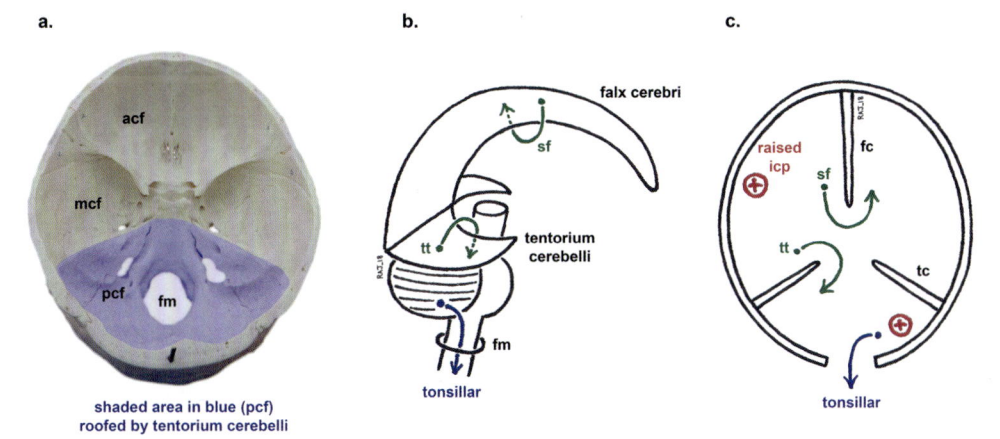

a.

acf
mcf
pcf fm

shaded area in blue (pcf)
roofed by tentorium cerebelli

b.

falx cerebri
sf
tt
tentorium cerebelli
fm
tonsillar

c.

raised icp
fc
sf
tt
tc
tonsillar

SAQ1 Base of skull and types of brain herniation. a. Base of skull and cranial fossae. b. and c. Types of brain herniation. **acf** anterior cranial fossa; **fc** falx cerebri; **fm** foramen magnum; **icp** intracranial pressure; **mcf** middle cranial fossa; **pcf** posterior cranial fossa; **sf** subfalcine; **tc** tentorium cerebelli; **tt** transtentorial.

a) **Where in the skull is the foramen magnum found? (1 mark)**
   Posterior cranial fossa; basilar part of the occipital bone

b) **Name four structures that pass through the foramen magnum (4 marks)**
   Osteo-ligamentous structures:
   - Tip of odontoid process
   - Ligaments (apical ligament, superior band of cruciate ligament, tectorial membrane)

   Neurovascular structures:
   - Lower end of medulla (with meninges)
   - Cerebellar tonsils (variant)
   - Spinal roots of CN 11 (either side, within subarachnoid space)
   - Vertebral arteries
   - Anterior and posterior spinal arteries (within subarachnoid space)

   (Anterior/posterior atlanto-occipital membranes attach to the margin of foramen magnum)

The osteo-ligamentous structures lie anterior to the alar ligaments, and the neurovascular structures lie posteriorly

Section 2: SAQs 1–12 (Answers)

c) **Name three types of brain herniation (3 marks)**
Subfalcine (cingulate), uncal (transtentorial) and tonsillar (cerebellar)
(Others: transcalvarial, central transtentorial, upward transtentorial)

> **CN 3 palsy:** dilated pupil (initially, loss of parasympathetic supply to pupil), 'down and out' (loss of supply to superior/medial inferior rectus and inferior oblique)
> **CN 6 palsy:** failure of lateral gaze/convergent squint (loss of supply to lateral rectus)

d) **Why may ocular features be a false-localising sign in brain injury causing cerebellar herniation? (2 marks)**
CN 3: may be compressed on margin of tentorium cerebelli by concurrent herniation of uncus
CN 6: has a long intracranial course, compressed by oedema in many intracranial locations

e) **Describe the pathophysiological changes of tonsillar (cerebellar) herniation (aka coning) (5 marks)**
Raised intracerebral pressure (ICP) results in raised mean arterial pressure (MAP) to maintain cerebral perfusion pressure (CPP) (**CPP = MAP − ICP**)
Eventually, raised ICP causes downward displacement of cerebellar tonsils
As they pass into the foramen magnum, the lower brainstem (medulla and pons) is compressed, with resulting dysfunction of the cardiac and respiratory centres
Initial pontine ischaemia results in a hyper-adrenergic state (to maintain brainstem perfusion)
Cushing's reflex (may only be present in one-third) suggests coning is imminent and describes:
- Hypertension (to maintain brainstem perfusion)
- Bradycardia (reflex baroreceptor activation due to hypertension +/− midbrain activation of the parasympathetic nervous system)
- Abnormal respiration (dysfunction of respiratory centre)

After herniation/neuronal death, the loss of spinal cord sympathetic discharge results in vasodilation, bradycardia and impaired contractility (with resultant cardiovascular instability)
Other dysfunction ensues:
- Pituitary ischaemia may result in diabetes insipidus (DI)
- Hypothalamic dysfunction may lead to loss of thermoregulation (compounded by vasodilation, reduced basal metabolic rate and hypothyroidism)
- Coagulopathy (catecholamine effects on platelets, hypothermia and release of plasminogen activator due to neuronal death)

f) **What hormone supplementation may be required in such patients if they are considered for brainstem death organ donation? (5 marks)**
Vasopressin (to maintain cardiovascular stability and for DI, noradrenaline is generally avoided)
Methylprednisolone (to reduce neurogenic pulmonary oedema)

Thyroid hormone (to maintain cardiac function)
Desmopressin (if DI persists despite the use of vasopressin)
Insulin (to combat hyperglycaemia resulting from catecholamine release, IV dextrose used to replace water in DI and steroids)

Section 2

SAQs 1–12 (Answers)

SAQ 2

Brachial Plexus and Axillary Block

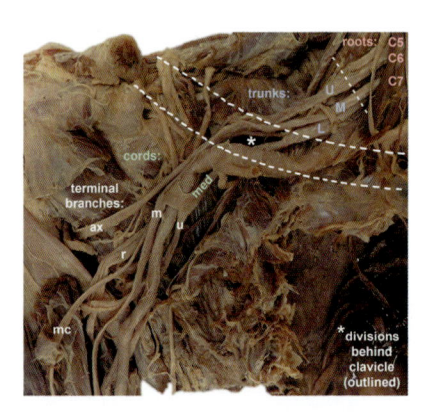

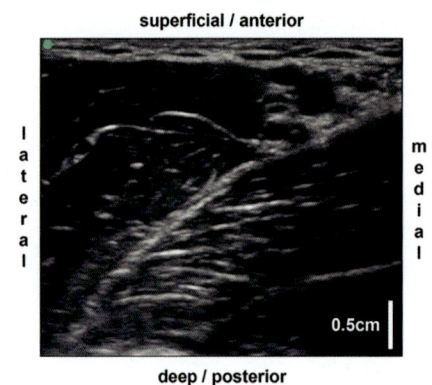

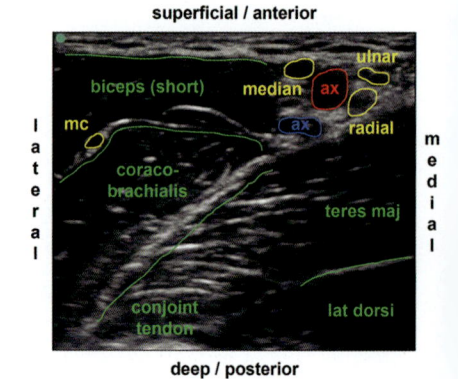

SAQ2 Brachial plexus. a. Dissection of brachial plexus. Divisions are behind clavicle; roots and trunks in neck (supraclavicular); cords (infraclavicular) and branches in axilla. b. Schematic of brachial plexus in same orientation as US image in c. **a** axillary artery; **ax** axillary; **L** lower; **M** middle; **m** median; **mc** musculocutaneous; **med** medial; **r** radial; **U** upper; **u** ulnar

SAQ 2: Brachial Plexus and Axillary Block

a) **What awake surgical procedures are permitted by the use of an axillary block? (2 marks)**
Procedures below the elbow: forearm, wrist and hand

b) **Name the nerves targeted when performing this block and where they are found* (4 marks)**
Musculocutaneous nerve (fascial plane between short head of biceps and coracobrachialis)
Median nerve (superolateral to the axillary artery, 9–12 o'clock position)
Ulnar nerve (inferomedial to axillary artery, beneath axillary vein, 2–3 o'clock position)
Radial nerve (deep to axillary artery, 4–6 o'clock position)

*These are typical positions, which vary between and within individuals – ultrasound is a dynamic process, scanning up and down the limb will confirm the identity of structures

c) **Regarding the musculocutaneous nerve:**
   i. **Why may it be missed during an axillary brachial plexus block?**
   Because it leaves the brachial plexus in the proximal axilla (therefore lies in a separate fascial plane at this level in 70% of the population, thus it should be blocked separately)
   ii. **What does it supply?**
   Motor supply: biceps, brachialis and coracobrachialis Sensory supply: lateral forearm (via its continuation as the lateral cutaneous nerve of forearm)
   iii. **How can a block of this nerve be supplemented? (3 marks)**
   By blocking the nerve at the level of the lateral epicondyle, between the lateral border of biceps and brachioradialis, where it can be seen on ultrasound adjacent to the cephalic vein

d) **What pattern of missed segment(s) is demonstrated in an inadequate axillary block? What areas are most likely to be spared in patients and why? What can be done to remedy this? (5 marks)**
Because the block is performed at the level of the terminal branches of the brachial plexus, missed segments demonstrate a nerve territory distribution (rather than dermatomal)
Medial side of forearm and (especially) arm, because:
- Intercostobrachial nerve (lateral cutaneous branch of T2) supplies skin over the medial proximal arm and is not blocked
- Medial cutaneous nerves of arm and forearm are branches of the medial cord of the brachial plexus in the axilla (before the ulnar nerve is given off) and therefore may be missed if not blocked separately

A subcutaneous injection of local anaesthetic in the medial proximal arm (or guided by ultrasound to target the medial cutaneous nerves of arm/forearm) can be performed

Section 2: SAQs 1–12 (Answers)

Brachial plexus block provides superior tourniquet coverage compared to distal nerve blocks (muscle ischaemia is the main problem) – this is an important consideration for upper limb surgery, in addition to covering the surgical site

e) **Describe a technique for performing an ultrasound-guided axillary brachial plexus block (6 marks)**

Consent
Stop before you block: confirm side and site
SLIMRAG*:

- Sterile procedure (wash hands, sterile gloves, sterile dressing pack)
- Light source/ultrasound
- IV access
- Monitoring (AAGBI minimum standard)
- Resuscitation drugs/equipment available
- Assistant (who is happy to assist with regional or general anaesthetic)
- General anaesthetic (ensure equipment/drugs available to convert if required)

*This acronym serves as an excellent aide memoire for the approach to almost any regional anaesthesia technique. It is taken from Shorthouse, Barker & Waldmann's *'SAQs for the Final FRCA'*.

Position the patient supine, upper limb abducted and externally rotated, elbow flexed at 90°
Clean the field with 0.5% chlorhexidine and allow to dry
High-frequency linear array transducer applied transversely across the axilla at the junction of biceps brachii and pectoralis major (with sterile cover and gel on probe)
Local anaesthetic to skin, then in-plane technique, blunt 22 G 50–80 mm block needle from lateral side of upper limb (can also be done out of plane)
Block the four nerves using sonoanatomy landmarks of axillary artery and vein
After negative aspiration slowly inject 25–30 ml of local anaesthetic, targeting each nerve
Can augment by block of intercostobrachial +/− medial cutaneous nerves of arm/forearm

Section 2 SAQs 1–12 (Answers)

SAQ 3

Bronchial Tree and Aspiration Pneumonia

a.

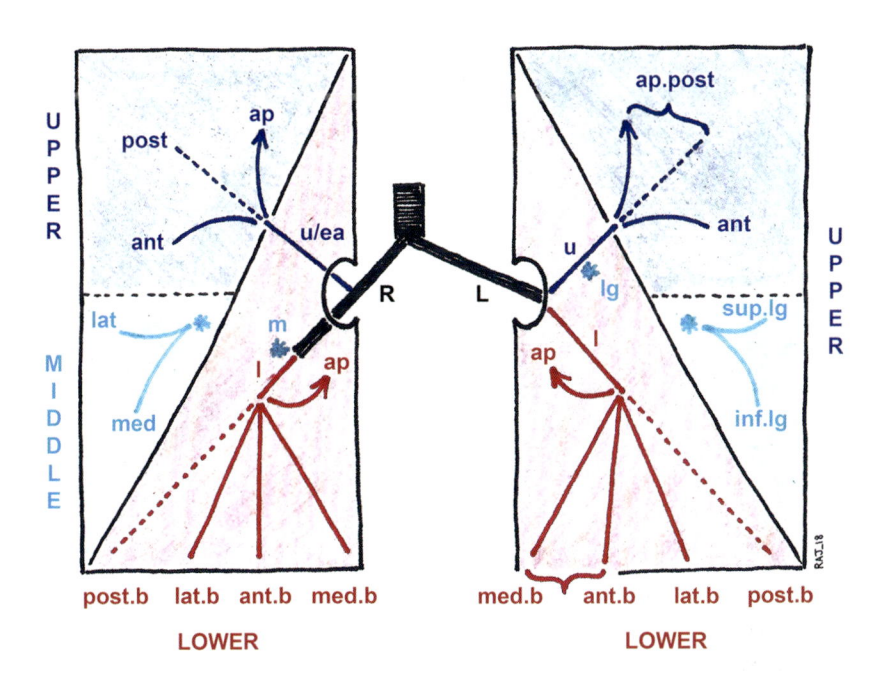

b.

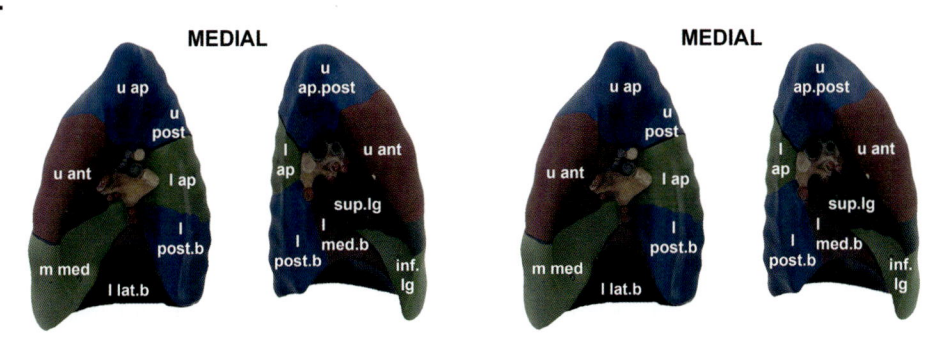

SAQ3 Bronchial tree. a. Schematic of bronchial tree and bronchopulmonary segments; note equivalence between lungs. b. Model of bronchopulmonary segments. **ant** anterior; **ap** apical; **ap.post** apico-posterior; **b** basal; **inf.lg** inferior lingular; **l** lower; **lat** lateral; **lg** lingular; **m** middle; **med** medial; **post** posterior; **sup.lg** superior lingular; **u/ea** upper/eparterial.

Section 2: SAQs 1–12 (Answers)

a) **Describe the structure of the respiratory tree (10 marks)**

The trachea bifurcates at the carina (plane of the sternal angle, T4–T4/5) into primary bronchi (left and right)

Right primary (or main) bronchus:
- Shorter, wider and more vertical
- Azygos vein arches forwards over the bronchus
- Divides into three secondary (lobar) bronchi: superior, middle and inferior
- N.B. Superior lobar bronchus (eparterial bronchus) is given off before the hilum of the lung

Left primary (or main) bronchus:
- Longer, narrower and more horizontal
- Passes beneath the arch of the aorta
- Passes immediately in front of (and indents) the oesophagus and descending thoracic aorta
- Divides into two secondary (lobar) bronchi: superior and inferior

The secondary bronchi divide into tertiary (segmental) bronchi
These each supply a bronchopulmonary segment:
- Right:
  - Upper lobe: apical, anterior, posterior
  - Middle lobe: medial, lateral
  - Lower lobe: apical, medial/lateral/anterior/posterior basal
- Left:
  - Upper lobe: apical, anterior*, posterior*, lingular (superior and inferior)
  - Lower lobe: apical, medial*/lateral/anterior**/posterior basal
- On average, the right side has 10 segments, left has 8–10

Tertiary (segmental) bronchi divide into many smaller bronchioles
Ultimately terminal bronchioles arise (1 mm diameter, no cartilage in wall)
These give rise to respiratory bronchioles (lose respiratory epithelium)
From these, alveolar ducts arise, and from these, alveolar sacs (which are clusters of alveoli)
In total there are 23 divisions of the bronchial tree
The first 17 form part of the conducting zone (finish at terminal bronchioles)
Generations 18–23 form part of the respiratory zone (start at respiratory bronchioles)

* and ** often conjoined, hence the variable (often fewer) number of bronchopulmonary segments quoted for the left lung

b) **Which segment(s) of which lung is most likely to be affected by aspiration of gastric contents (3 marks)**

More likely on right (as right main bronchus is shorter, wider and more vertical)
Depends on position:

- Supine: apical segment of right lower lobe
- Standing/sitting: posterior basal segment of right lower lobe
- Lying on right: right middle lobe or posterior segment of right upper lobe

c) **Describe the pathophysiology of aspiration pneumonitis (3 marks)**
Large particles cause acute airway obstruction +/− lobar collapse and atelectasis
Initial changes due to acute inflammatory response resulting from chemical irritation (aspiration pneumonitis due to haemorrhagic tracheobronchitis and pulmonary oedema)
The most likely complication is acute respiratory distress syndrome (ARDS) (infection may or may not result)

d) **How do you manage aspiration in a patient with a supraglottic airway device? (4 marks)**
Call for help and ask surgeon to stop (only restart if patient stable +/− emergency surgery)
FiO_2 to 1
Move patient to left lateral position (if possible, head down)
Suction oropharynx, down lumen (if a second-generation supraglottic airway device (SAD) is being used, suction down the gastric port +/− pass a narrow bore NG tube to aspirate/decompress the stomach)
If major airway contamination/desaturation: consider intubation, positive pressure ventilation, bronchoalveolar lavage, bronchodilators, ITU post-op
If minimal: ensure SAD correctly placed, airway is clear and patient is adequately anaesthetised, then CXR in recovery (only antibiotics if subsequently develops infection)

Section 2
SAQs 1–12 (Answers)

SAQ 4
Epidural Space and Epidural

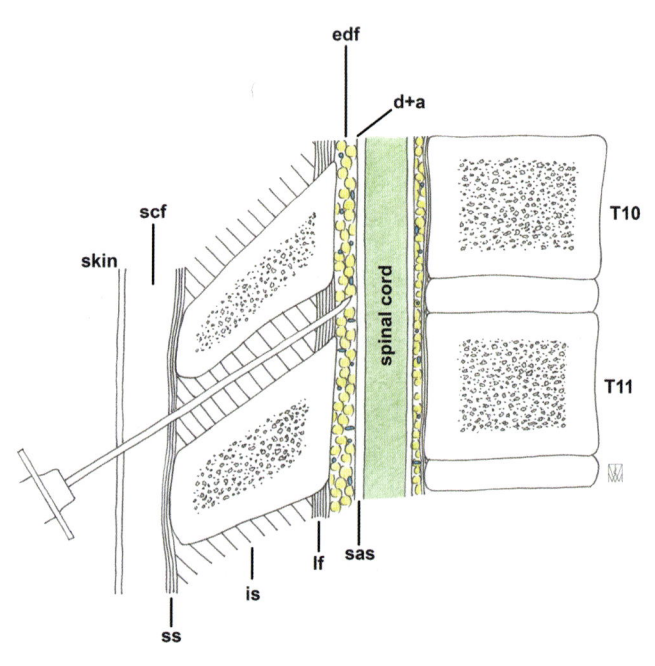

SAQ4 Epidural space. Schematic to demonstrate the layers traversed during epidural block. **d+a** dura & arachnoid; **edf** epidural fat; **is** interspinous ligament; **lf** ligamentum flavum; **sas** subarachnoid space; **scf** subcutaneous fat; **ss** supraspinous ligament.

a) Describe the boundaries of the epidural space (4 marks)
   Extends from the foramen magnum superiorly to the sacral hiatus (sacrococcygeal membrane) inferiorly
   Anteriorly: the vertebral bodies and intervertebral discs, covered by the posterior longitudinal ligament
   Laterally: the pedicles and the intervertebral foramina
   Posteriorly: the laminae of the vertebral arches, the capsules of facet joints and ligamenta flava

SAQ 4: Epidural Space and Epidural

b) **List the contents of the epidural space (6 marks)**
   Dural sheath/sac and contents (arachnoid mater, subarachnoid space and CSF, pia mater, spinal cord/spinal nerve roots and spinal arteries/veins)
   Spinal nerve roots (within a sleeve of dura/arachnoid)
   Filum terminale (beyond the termination of the dural sac at S2)
   Vessels:
   - (Anterior and posterior) radicular arteries
   - Internal vertebral venous plexus of Batson

   Lymphatics
   Loose areolar tissue* (fat content varies in direct proportion to the rest of the body)
   Connective tissue**

   *Apparently this is not uniform in distribution and exists in bands at the levels of intervertebral foramina
   **A median fold of dura has been reported and would explain the occasional unilateral effect of epidural analgesia)

c) **What structures does the Tuohy needle pass through when performing a midline epidural? (5 marks)**
   Skin
   Subcutaneous tissue/superficial fascia
   Supraspinous ligament
   Interspinous ligament
   Ligamentum flavum (ligamenta flava lie either side of the midline, between laminae of two adjacent vertebrae, but may be fused in the midline)

d) **What are the benefits of epidural analgesia after laparotomy for malignant disease? (5 marks)**
   Short term:
   - Lower pain scores
   - Reduce opioid consumption (and associated side effects: respiratory depression, nausea/vomiting, immunosuppression)
   - Reduced stress response, sympathetic activation and immunosuppression
   - Lower transfusion requirements
   - Reduced incidence of respiratory failure and postoperative pneumonia
   - Reduced incidence of DVT/PE

   Long term:
   - Reduced metastatic spread

Section 2 SAQs 1–12 (Answers)

SAQ 5: Femoral Triangle and Fascia Iliaca Block

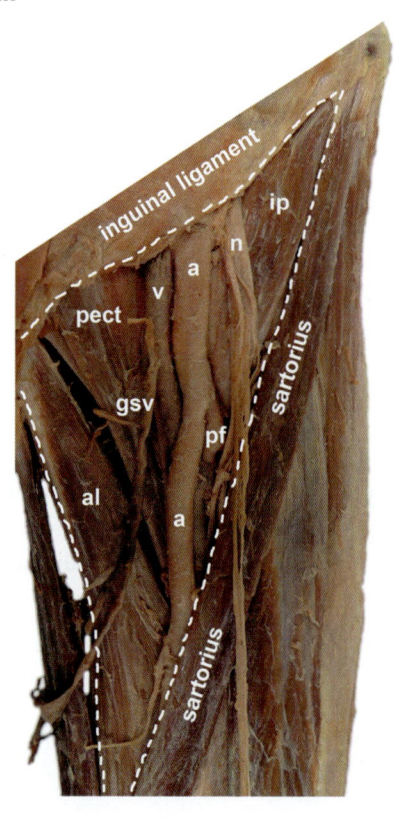

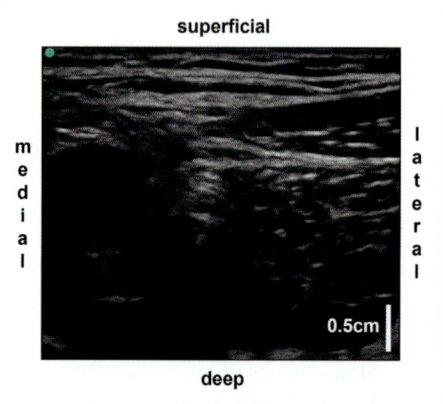

a.

b.

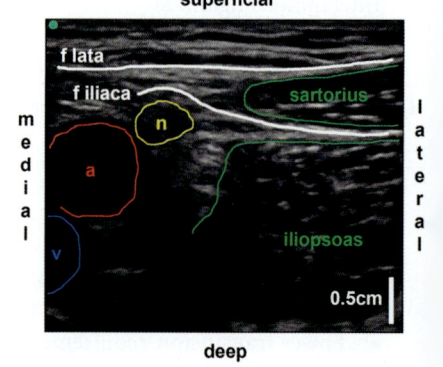

SAQ5 Femoral triangle. a. Dissection of femoral triangle. b. US scan of groin; note positions of fascia lata and fascia iliaca. **a** femoral artery; **al** adductor longus; **f iliaca** fascia iliaca; **f lata** fascia lata; **gsv** great saphenous vein; **ip** iliopsoas; **n** femoral nerve; **pect** pectineus; **pf** profunda femoris artery; **v** femoral vein.

a) Describe the boundaries and contents of the femoral triangle (6 marks)
   Boundaries:
   - Superior: inguinal ligament
   - Lateral: medial border of sartorius
   - Medial: medial border of adductor longus

- Roof: fascia lata (and cribriform fascia at saphenous opening), skin/subcutaneous tissue
- Floor: iliacus, psoas major, pectineus, adductor longus

Contents:
- Femoral nerve
- Femoral sheath, containing:
  - Femoral artery (and branches)
  - Femoral vein (and tributaries, including long saphenous vein)
  - Femoral canal (containing lymphatics/deep inguinal lymph nodes, including node of Cloquet)

b) **What is a fascia iliaca block? (2 marks)**
   It is a compartment block where local anaesthetic is deposited into the plane between the deep fascia overlying the iliacus muscle, where several branches of the lumbar plexus are found (femoral nerve courses through a pocket of the fascia iliaca)
   Therefore, a large volume of local anaesthetic is required (e.g. 30 ml)

N.B. Obturator nerve (L2–4, supplying hip, medial/adductor compartment of thigh and skin of medial thigh/knee) – block is described in fascia iliaca technique, but rarely occurs as the nerve emerges on the medial side of psoas major

c) **Describe the borders of the fascia iliaca compartment and nerves affected by the block (6 marks)**
   Borders:
- Anterior: fascia iliaca
- Posterior: anterior surface of iliacus and psoas major/their conjoint tendon
- Medial: linea terminalis/pelvic brim
- Lateral: inner lip of iliac crest

Nerves:
- Femoral nerve (L2–4): supplies hip, anterior/extensor compartment of this, skin of anterior thigh/medial leg and medial foot to first MTPJ
- Lateral cutaneous nerve of thigh (L2–3): supplies skin of anterolateral thigh

d) **Describe how you would perform a fascia iliaca block (6 marks)**
   Consent
   Stop before you block: confirm side and site
   SLIMRAG:
- Sterile procedure (wash hands, sterile gloves, sterile dressing pack)
- Light source/ultrasound
- IV access
- Monitoring (AAGBI minimum standard)
- Resuscitation drugs/equipment available
- Assistant (who is happy to assist with regional or general anaesthetic)
- General anaesthetic (ensure equipment/drugs available to convert if required)

- Position the patient lying, with proximal thigh exposed
- Clean the field with 0.5% chlorhexidine and allow to dry
- Needle insertion 2 cm below the junction of medial two-thirds and lateral one-third of the inguinal ligament
- High-frequency linear array ultrasound probe with sterile cover and gel
- Out of plane technique probably better at allowing the operator to ensure needle is deep to the fascia iliaca and avoid nerve or vascular injury by the needle
- Local anaesthetic to skin, pass short bevel 50-mm needle through fascia lata and fascia iliaca, at an angle of 45° (directed cranially)
- After negative aspiration, slowly inject 30 ml local anaesthetic* (e.g. 0.25% levo-bupivacaine), confirming negative aspiration after every 5-ml injection (+/− distal pressure)
- Fluid-filled space created deep to fascia iliaca/superficial to iliacus muscle, as it increases in size during the injection, fluid travels cephalic beneath the fascia and contacts the nerves mentioned above

*Confirm the safe dose pre-procedure – this block is often performed in cases of fractured neck of femur where patients may have a low body weight, so care with dosing is advised

Section 2 — SAQs 1–12 (Answers)

SAQ 6

Internal Jugular Vein and Cannulation

a.

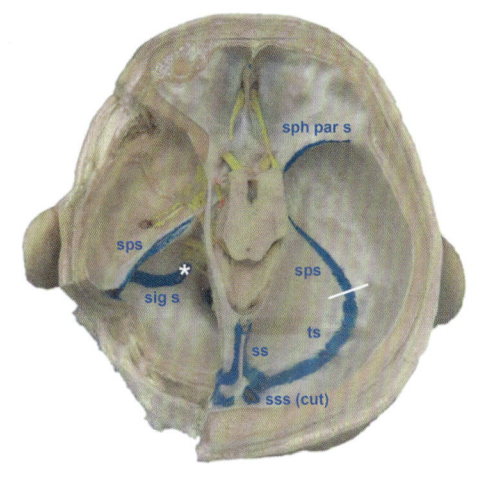

b.

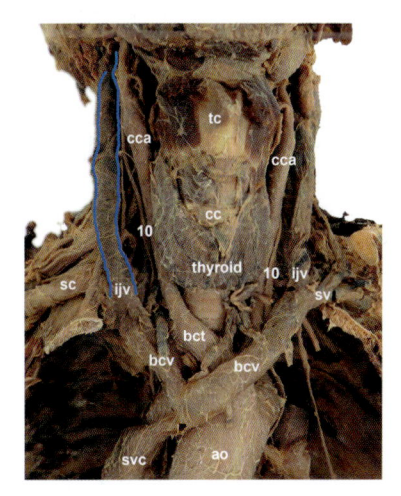

c.

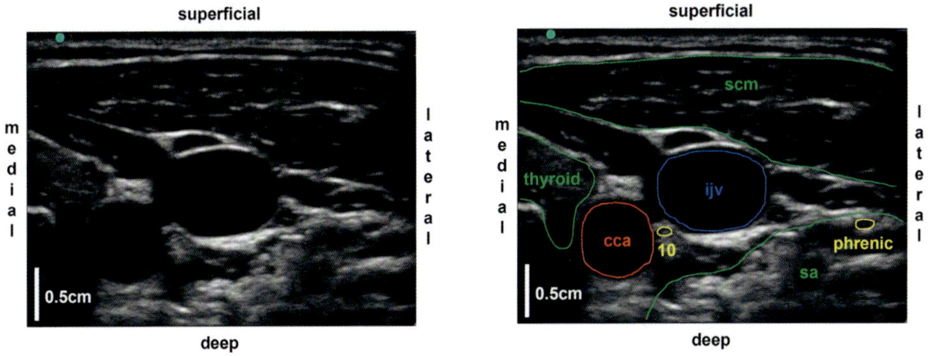

SAQ6 Internal jugular vein. a. Dural venous sinuses. b. Dissection of neck. c. US image of IJV and surrounding structures. **10** vagus nerve; **ao** aorta; **bct** brachiocephalic trunk; **bcv** brachiocephalic vein; **cc** cricoid cartilage; **cca** common carotid artery; **ijv** internal jugular vein; **sa** scalenus anterior; **sc** subclavian artery; **scm** sternocleidomastoid; **sig s** sigmoid sinus; **sph par s** sphenoparietal sinus; **sps** superior petrosal sinus; **ss** straight sinus; **sss** superior sagittal sinus; **sv** subclavian vein; **svc** superior vena cava; **tc** thyroid cartilage; **ts** transverse sinus.

Section 2: SAQs 1–12 (Answers)

a) **Describe the origin, course and termination of the internal jugular vein (IJV). Make specific reference to its relationship with the carotid artery (5 marks)**

Emerges through the posterior compartment of the jugular foramen as a continuation of the sigmoid sinus

(Origin sometimes described as the point where it combines with the inferior petrosal sinus)

Lies posterior to the internal carotid artery at the base of the skull (on the transverse process of the atlas)

As it passes inferiorly in the neck, it comes to lie on the lateral side of the internal carotid artery

In the lower neck, the IJV typically lies anterior/anterolateral to the common carotid artery

Terminates behind the medial end of the clavicle, joining with the subclavian vein to form the brachiocephalic vein

b) **Describe features that distinguish the jugular venous pulse (JVP) from the carotid pulse (5 marks)**

JVP is impalpable

JVP has a complex waveform

JVP fills from the top (if IJV occluded)

JVP demonstrates the hepatojugular reflux (JVP will transiently rise with hepatic pressure)

JVP moves with respiration (normally decreasing on inspiration and rising in expiration)

c) **List five indications for cannulating the IJV (5 marks)**

Monitoring CVP/RV function/intravascular volume status

Administration of drugs that cannot be given peripherally (vasoactive drugs/inotropes, vaso-irritant drugs, e.g. potassium/amiodarone, total parenteral nutrition (TPN), some cytotoxic drugs)

Blood sampling due to poor vascular access

Insertion of pulmonary artery catheter (or its introducer sheath for large-bore IV access +/− rapid fluid administration)

Haemodialysis/haemofiltration

Transvenous cardiac pacing

Aspiration of air embolus from right-hand side of the heart

Jugular venous bulb saturation measurement

d) **List five complications of cannulating the IJV (5 marks)**

Due to needle:
- Carotid artery puncture (+/− bleeding, dissection, embolus)
- Pneumothorax (or haemothorax)
- Thoracic duct injury (+/− chylothorax)
- Nerve injury (e.g. CN 10, recurrent laryngeal, phrenic)

Due to line:
- Arrhythmia
- Air embolism
- Thrombosis/embolism (+/− vessel stenosis)
- Infection
- Cardiac tamponade/haemopericardium
- Anaphylaxis has been reported from chlorhexidine-impregnated catheters

Section 2 — SAQs 1–12 (Answers)

SAQ 7 — Intercostal Space and Chest Drain/Procedures

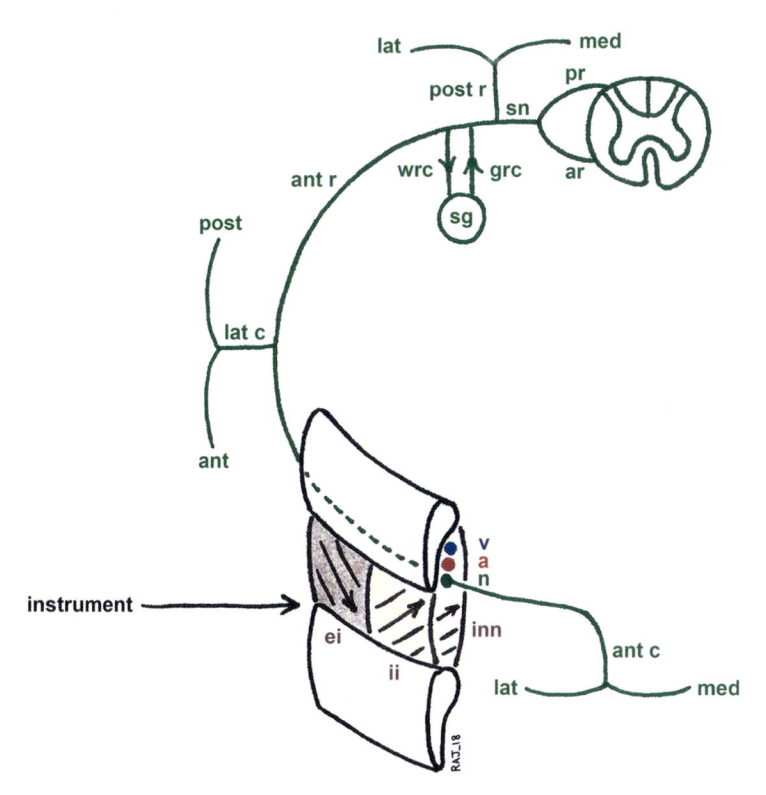

SAQ7 Intercostal space. Schematic of spinal nerve and intercostal space. **ant** anterior; **ant c** anterior cutaneous branch; **ant r** anterior ramus; **ar** anterior root; **ei** external intercostals; **grc** grey ramus communicans; **ii** internal intercostals; **inn** innermost intercostals; **lat** lateral; **lat c** lateral cutaneous branch; **med** medial; **post** posterior; **post r** posterior ramus; **pr** posterior root; **sg** sympathetic ganglion; **sn** spinal nerve; **wrc** white ramus communicans.

a) Name the tissue layers traversed during insertion of an intercostal (chest) drain (5 marks)
Skin
Superficial fascia
External intercostal muscle
Internal intercostal muscle
Innermost intercostal muscle
Endothoracic fascia
Parietal pleura

b) **Name and describe the muscles of the intercostal space (6 marks)**
   External intercostal:
   - Outermost layer, fibres pass downwards and forwards from sharp inferior border of rib
   - Extends from tubercle of rib (posteriorly) to costochondral junction (anteriorly)
   - From the costochondral junction to the margin of the sternum, the muscle layer is replaced by the anterior intercostal membrane

   Internal intercostal:
   - Middle layer, fibres pass downwards and backwards from the costal groove
   - Extends from the margin of the sternum (anteriorly) to the angle of the rib (posteriorly)
   - From the angle of the rib to the tubercle, the muscle is replaced by the posterior intercostal membrane

   Innermost layer:
   - Discontinuous; separated into three parts:
     1. Sternocostalis (aka transversus thoracis, anteriorly)
     2. Innermost intercostals (laterally: the major part of the inner layer)
     3. Subcostalis (posteriorly)
   - Muscle fibres from the anterior (1) and posterior (3) part of this layer cross more than one intercostal space

c) **With the aid of a diagram, describe the structure of a spinal nerve from the T2–6 level, after it has emerged from the vertebral column. State where it lies in the intercostal space (6 marks)**
   31 pairs of spinal nerves, emerge from the intervertebral foramen (anterior and posterior rami of S1–4 emerge through anterior and posterior sacral foramina respectively)
   The thoracic intercostal nerves (T2–6) divide into anterior and posterior divisions (rami)
   The posterior ramus supplies only the muscles of the back (including erector spinae) and overlying skin to a hand's breadth either side of the midline
   The anterior ramus passes forwards between the middle and innermost intercostal layers
   At the angle of the rib, a collateral branch is given off, which runs forwards in the lower part of the space and provides supply to the intercostal muscles, parietal pleura, periosteum and the periphery of the diaphragm (T7–11 only, not T2–6)
   The main trunk of the nerve continues in the intercostal space and is mostly sensory to skin, giving a lateral cutaneous branch at the midaxillary line and ending as an anterior cutaneous branch at the edge of the sternum

d) **Name three procedures in anaesthesia, other than intercostal drain insertion, which make use of the intercostal space (3 marks)**
Cannula decompression of tension pneumothorax
Regional anaesthesia (intercostal nerve and interpleural block)
Ultrasound (echocardiography and lung ultrasound in intensive care)
(Non-anaesthesia: pleural aspiration (draining fluid/air, sampling fluid), thoracotomy, lung biopsy)

Section 2 — SAQs 1–12 (Answers)

SAQ 8 — Lumbar Plexus and Lumbar Plexus Block

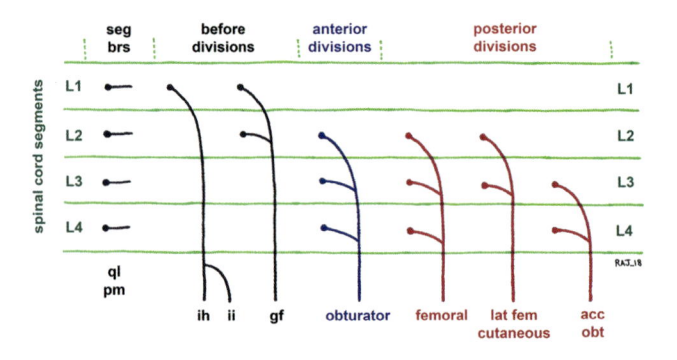

a.

b.

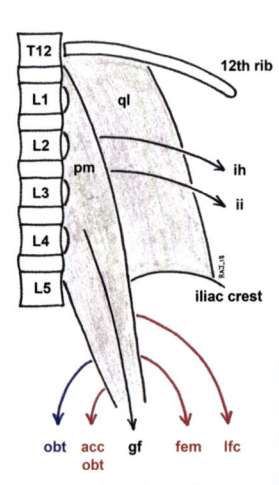

SAQ8 Lumbar plexus. a. and b. Schematics of lumbar plexus. **acc obt** accessory obturator; **fem** femoral; **gf** genitofemoral; **ih** iliohypogastric; **ii** ilioinguinal; **lfc** lateral femoral cutaneous; **obt** obturator; **pm** psoas major; **ql** quadratus lumborum; **seg brs** segmental branches.

a) Which nerve root contributes to the lumbar plexus, in what muscle is it formed and where is the muscle found? (4 marks)
From the anterior rami of L1–4 (sometimes with a contribution from T12)
It is formed within the substance of psoas major muscle (posterior third)
Psoas major lies between the 12th rib and iliac crest on the posterior abdominal wall, anterior to the lumbar transverse processes, and lateral to the lumbar vertebral bodies/intervertebral discs and foramina

b) Name the branches of the lumbar plexus and their respective root value (6 marks)
Iliohypogastric nerve (L1 +/− T12)
Ilioinguinal* (L1)
Genitofemoral (L1–2)
Lateral cutaneous nerve of the thigh (L2–3)
Obturator nerve** (L2–4)
Femoral nerve (L2–4)

*The collateral branch of the iliohypogastric nerve
**An accessory obturator nerve is also present in around 25%

c) **Name indications and contraindications for a lumbar plexus block (5 marks)**
Indications:
- Analgesia of the ipsilateral lower limb (hip, femur, knee)

Absolute contraindications:
- Patient refusal
- Local anaesthetic allergy
- Local sepsis/infection (puncture site or within psoas compartment)
- Coagulopathy

Relative contraindications:
- Systemic sepsis (particularly for catheter placement)
- Fixed cardiac output (due to the risk of epidural/subarachnoid spread)

d) **What complications of regional anaesthesia are pertinent to lumbar plexus blockade? (5 marks)**
From needle:
- Direct trauma to nerves of the lumbar plexus/intraneural injection
- Dural puncture
- Trauma to retroperitoneal structures/abdominal viscera (e.g. kidney, ureteric injury)
- Retroperitoneal haematoma
- Psoas abscess

From incorrect placement of local anaesthetic:
- Epidural/intrathecal spread of local anaesthetic

From local anaesthetic:
- Hypotension
- Intravascular injection/local anaesthetic systemic toxicity (psoas compartment is highly vascular and muscle tissue demonstrates rapid drug absorption)

Section 2

SAQs 1–12 (Answers)

SAQ 9

Oesophagus

a.

b.

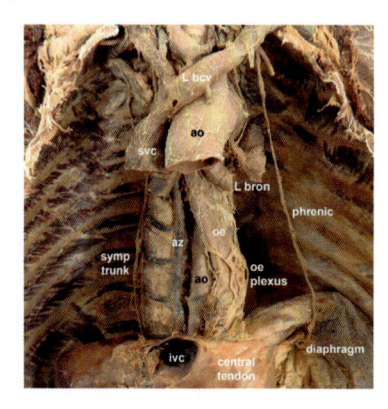

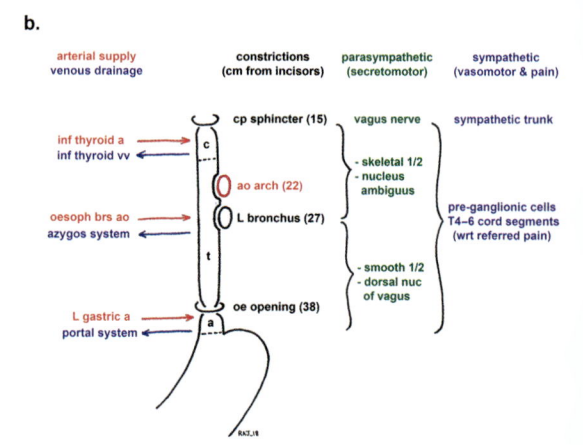

SAQ9 Oesophagus. a. Dissection of posterior mediastinum to demonstrate oesophagus and relationships. **b.** Schematic of oesophagus (cervical, thoracic, abdominal) showing blood supply, nerve supply and constrictions. **ao** aorta; **az** azygos vein; **bcv** brachiocephalic vein; **cp sphincter** cricopharyngeal sphincter; **ivc** inferior vena cava; **L bron** left bronchus; **oe** oesophagus; **svc** superior vena cava; **symp trunk** sympathetic trunk.

a) **Describe the neurovascular supply of the oesophagus (9 marks)**
   Nerve supply:
   - Motor: CN 10*, recurrent laryngeal branches for upper third and vagal plexi for rest
   - Sensory: pain fibres run with both parasympathetic (CN 10) and sympathetic fibres** (T2–6, from the middle and lower cervical ganglia)
   - Secretomotor: CN 10

   Arterial supply:
   - Cervical portion: oesophageal branches of inferior thyroid artery (arise from the thyrocervical trunk – third branch of the first part of the subclavian artery***)
   - Thoracic portion: oesophageal branches of thoracic aorta
   - Abdominal portion: oesophageal branches of left gastric artery (from the celiac trunk)

   Venous drainage via oesophageal veins to:
   - Cervical portion: inferior thyroid vein (draining to brachiocephalic vein; *systemic*)
   - Thoracic portion: azygos vein (draining to SVC; *systemic*)
   - Abdominal portion: oesophageal tributaries of left gastric vein (draining to *portal* vein)

SAQ 9: Oesophagus

> *Vagal fibres from the nucleus ambiguus supply upper third striated muscle of the oesophagus, fibres from dorsal motor nucleus for lower visceral muscle
> **This explains the referred pain of oesophagitis – retrosternal dermatomes T2–6
> ***In 25%, arises directly from the third part of the subclavian artery

b) **List the relations of the thoracic oesophagus (4 marks)**
   Anterior: trachea, left main bronchus, pericardium/left atrium, (left) recurrent laryngeal nerve, anterior vagal trunk
   Posterior: vertebral bodies, thoracic duct (crossing to the left at T5), descending thoracic aorta, connections to (accessory)/hemiazygos vein, posterior vagal trunk
   Right: pleura, **azygos vein******
   Left: pleura, **arch of aorta******, thoracic duct (above T5)

> ****The blue arch is right, the red arch is left

c) **What anaesthetic monitoring devices are placed in the oesophagus and what do they measure? (3 marks)**
   Oesophageal Doppler (cardiac output)
   Transoesophageal echocardiography probe (cardiac structure and function, fluid filling)
   Oesophageal temperature probe (core temperature)
   Oesophageal contractility (depth of anaesthesia)

d) **What features, of the distal oesophagus and surrounding structures, form the 'physiological sphincter' of the lower oesophagus to reduce reflux of gastric contents? (4 marks)**
   Tonic contraction of circular smooth muscle in the lower oesophagus
   Fibres of the right crus of the diaphragm surround the lower oesophagus
   Longitudinal folds of oesophageal mucosa occluding the central lumen
   The oesophagus enters the stomach at an acute angle
   The terminal 2–3 cm of the oesophagus are below the diaphragm (raised intra-abdominal pressure compresses the oesophagus causing a flap-valve effect)
   N.B. Gravity is also a contributing factor when upright – hence why patients may experience gastro-oesophageal reflux disease predominantly when lying down

SAQs 1–12 (Answers)

SAQ 10: Pituitary Gland and Transsphenoidal Approach

a.

b.

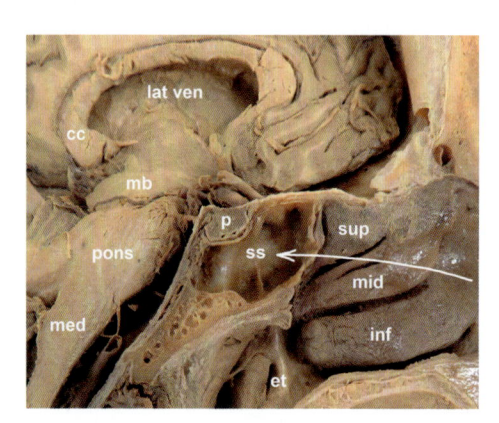

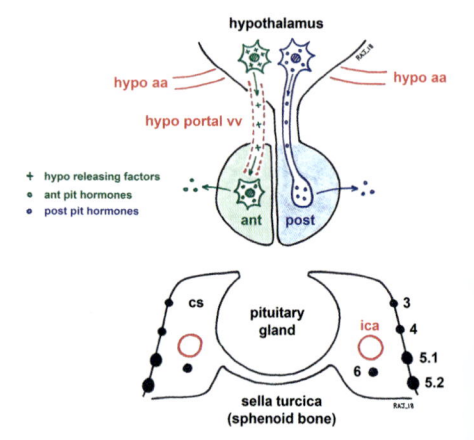

SAQ10 Pituitary gland. a. Median section. Arrow shows transsphenoidal approach to pituitary gland. b. Schematic of pituitary gland and cavernous sinus. **cc** corpus callosum; **cs** cavernous sinus; **et** Eustachian tube; **hypo** hypophyseal; **ica** internal carotid artery; **inf** inferior concha; **lat ven** lateral ventricle; **mb** midbrain; **med** medulla; **mid** middle concha; **p** pituitary; **ss** sphenoidal sinus; **sup** superior concha.

a) **Describe the anatomy of the pituitary gland and its relations (8 marks)**

An endocrine gland at the base of the brain, composed of a (larger) anterior lobe and (smaller) posterior lobe, separated by a pars intermedia

Located in the pituitary fossa (or sella turcica – the 'Turkish saddle'), a depression in the sphenoid bone and the central portion of the middle cranial fossa

The roof of the sella turcica is formed by a fold dura (the diaphragma sellae); a small perforation allows the pituitary stalk to pass through in continuity with the hypothalamus (above) and posterior pituitary (below)

Relations:
- Lateral: cavernous sinus, containing the internal carotid artery and CN 6 (with CN 3, CN 4, CN 5.1 and 5.2 lying in the lateral wall of the cavernous sinus)
- Superior: optic chiasma (anteriorly), hypothalamus and, above that, the third ventricle
- Anterior/inferior: sphenoidal air sinus
- Posterior: midbrain and pons

SAQ 10: Pituitary Gland and Transsphenoidal Approach

b) **What is the hypothalamo-hypophyseal portal venous system? (2 marks)**

Microcirculation connecting the hypothalamus with the pituitary to expedite transport and exchange of hormones between the hypothalamus and anterior pituitary

Blood from the superior hypophyseal (pituitary) arteries supplies the hypothalamus where they form a primary capillary plexus receiving the hypothalamic hormones

Blood then drains (by hypophyseal portal veins) to a secondary plexus in the anterior pituitary, where the hypothalamic hormones affect their target cells (in the anterior pituitary)

These capillaries are highly permeable to facilitate the exchange of these hormones

c) **What features of acromegaly are relevant to the conduct of general anaesthesia? (5 marks)**

Airway:
- Up to 70% have obstructive sleep apnoea (OSA) due to generalised hypertrophy/oedema of upper airway mucosa
- This, combined with development of macrognathia and macroglossia can make bag-mask ventilation and intubation more difficult

Respiratory:
- Proximal muscle weakness and potential OSA increase risk of postoperative respiratory failure

Cardiac:
- Hypertension and left ventricular hypertrophy (LVH) lead to increased risk of cardiac ischaemia and failure

Endocrine:
- Multiple endocrine abnormalities can occur, in particular diabetes mellitus, hyper-/hypothyroidism and adrenal insufficiency

Other:
- Venous cannulation may be difficult due to excess soft tissue

d) **What is the transsphenoidal approach to the pituitary gland? Name the main advantages and complications (5 marks)**

Transsphenoidal approach:
- Elevate the mucosa from the posterior nasal septum (requires fracture/removal of the anterior bony septum, the posterior part is removed but preserved for closure)
- Through this opening enter the sphenoidal air sinus and, from here, enter the pituitary fossa

Advantages:
- Improved access
- Avoidance of craniotomy: reduced surgical trauma/pain, cosmetic benefit
- Reduced blood loss

Complications:
- Haemorrhage
- Cranial nerve injury (in particular visual deficit)
- Persistent CSF leak
- Hormonal (panhypopituitarism or transient DI)
- Ischaemic stroke (due to vasospasm)

Section 2 SAQs 1–12 (Answers)

SAQ 11: Popliteal Fossa and Block

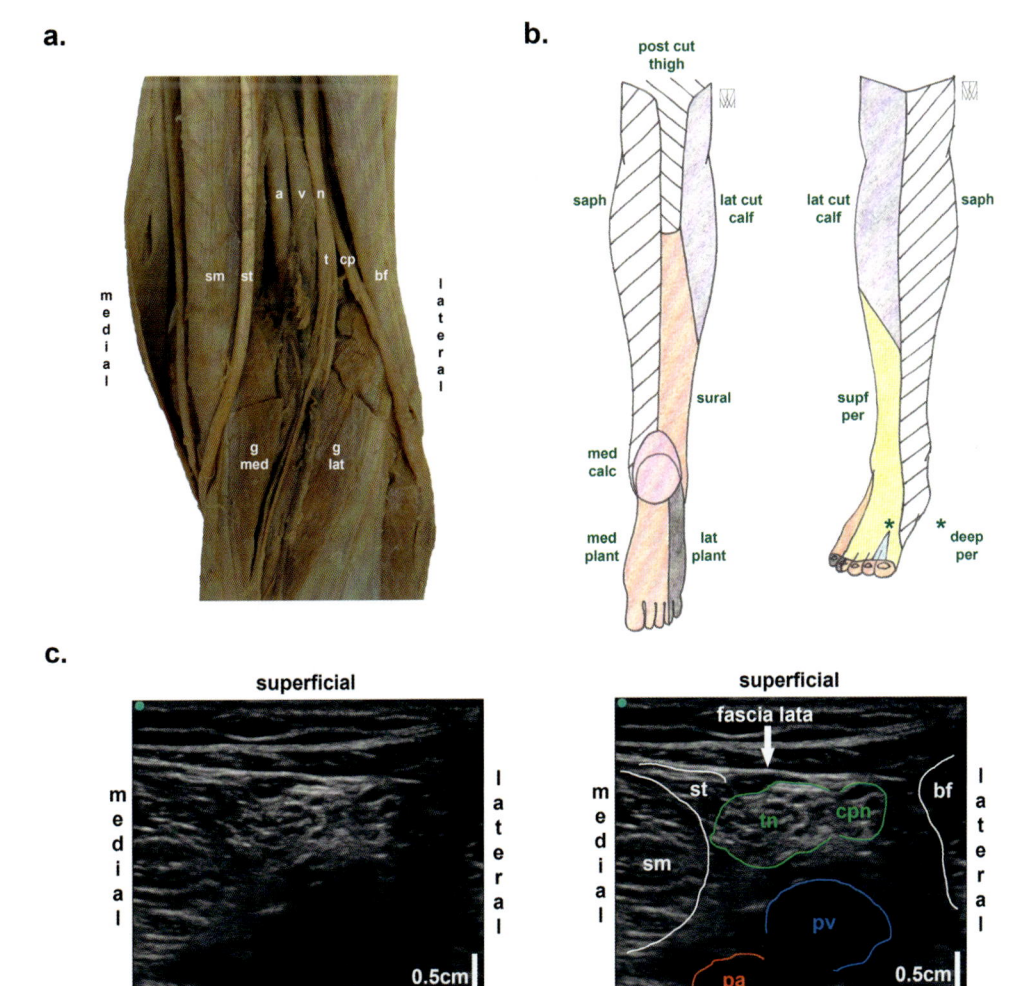

a.

b.

c.

SAQ11 a. **Dissection of popliteal fossa**. b. Peripheral nerve distribution – blocked branches of the tibial and common peroneal nerves are coloured; nerves that escape the block are shown hatched. c. US image of the popliteal fossa. **a** popliteal artery; **bf** biceps femoris; **cp** common peroneal nerve; **cpn** common peroneal nerve; **deep per** deep peroneal; **g lat** gastrocnemius (lateral head); **g med** gastrocnemius (medial head); **lat cut calf** lateral cutaneous nerve of calf; **lat plant** lateral plantar; **med calc** medial calcaneal; **med plant** medial plantar; **n** tibial nerve; **pa** popliteal artery; **post cut thigh** posterior cutaneous nerve of thigh; **pv** popliteal vein; **saph** saphenous nerve; **sm** semimembranosus; **st** semitendinosus; **supf per** superficial peroneal; **t** tibial nerve; **tn** tibial nerve; **v** popliteal vein.

Section 2: SAQs 1–12 (Answers)

a) **What are the indications for a popliteal fossa block? (3 marks)**
Surgical procedures below the knee:
- Foot/ankle surgery (corrective, debridement/amputation, Achilles tendon repair)
- Interventional radiology to revascularise lower limb below the knee
- Other: sural nerve biopsy, short saphenous vein (SSV) stripping
- (Rescue) analgesia for leg/ankle/foot pain (e.g. trauma or postoperative)

b) **Describe the anatomy of the popliteal fossa (5 marks)**
Boundaries:
- **Superomedial:** the '**semi**' muscles (semimembranosus and semitendinosus)
- **Superolateral:** medial border of biceps femoris
- **Inferomedial:** gastrocnemius (medial head)
- **Inferolateral:** gastrocnemius (lateral head)
- Roof: fascia lata
- Floor (proximal to distal): popliteal surface of femur, capsule of knee joint, popliteus

Contents (superficial to deep):
- Short saphenous vein (pierces roof of popliteal fossa and drains into popliteal vein)
- Tibial and common peroneal nerves*
- Popliteal vein
- Popliteal artery
- Popliteal lymph nodes and fat pack the rest of the fossa

*The terminal branches of the sciatic nerve – the bifurcation is typically at the apex of the popliteal fossa, but it can occur as far proximally as the gluteal region

c) **Describe the cutaneous innervation of the sciatic nerve below the knee (6 marks)**
Tibial (L4–S3):
- Lower half of lateral calf and lateral border of foot, including little toe (sural nerve)
- Plantar surface of foot (medial and lateral plantar nerves)
- Heel (medial calcaneal branches)

Common peroneal/fibular (L4–S2):
- Upper half of lateral calf (lateral cutaneous nerve of calf)
- Lower anterolateral calf and dorsum of foot (superficial peroneal nerve)
- First web space (deep peroneal nerve)
- (N.B. Also contributes to the sural nerve via a communicating branch)

d) **Describe a technique for performing a popliteal fossa block (6 marks)**
Consent
Stop before you block: confirm side and site**
SLIMRAG:
- Sterile procedure (wash hands, sterile gloves, sterile dressing pack)
- Light source/ultrasound
- IV access
- Monitoring (AAGBI minimum standard)

SAQ 11: Popliteal Fossa and Block

- Resuscitation drugs/equipment available
- Assistant (who is happy to assist with regional or general anaesthetic)
- General anaesthetic: ensure equipment/drugs available to convert if required

Position: supine (flex knee to 30°) or lateral (block limb uppermost), occasionally prone

Locate skin crease at popliteal fossa and clean skin of distal lateral thigh with 0.5% chlorhexidine (allow to dry)

High-frequency linear array ultrasound probe with sterile cover and gel to identify sciatic nerve bifurcation (typically 5–10 cm proximal to the popliteal skin crease)

In-plane technique, 80–100 mm short bevel regional block needle

Apply local anaesthetic to skin then insert from lateral side (anterior to tendon of biceps femoris)

After negative aspiration, slowly inject 15–20 ml of local anaesthetic, aiming for perineurial deposition of local anaesthetic around the division of the sciatic nerve, confirming negative aspiration after every 5-ml injection

**Particularly important as the patient is often turned either lateral or prone to perform the block, increasing risk of wrong site block

Block tips...

A peripheral nerve stimulator may be used to guide nerve localisation; however, the sciatic nerve contains sensory nerve fibres at this level – this may lead to false negative results if relying on eliciting a motor response

The popliteal vein is easily compressed by pressure from the ultrasound transducer, and care must be taken to ensure that the vein has not been cannulated – this is achieved by visualising the needle tip, negative aspiration, 5-ml aliquots of local anaesthetic, visualisation of local anaesthetic spread and monitoring the patient for signs of local anaesthetic toxicity

Section 2

SAQs 1–12 (Answers)

SAQ 12

Trachea and Tracheostomy

a.

* location of emergency airway (cricothyroidotomy)

** location of tracheostomy (2nd/3rd tracheal rings)

b.

1. investing 3. carotid sheath
2. pre-tracheal 4. pre-vertebral

c.

SAQ12 Trachea. a. Schematic of trachea and surrounding structures. b. Schematic of transverse sections through neck at commencement (C6) and termination (T4) of trachea. c. US images of IJV and surrounding structures. **aj** anterior jugular; **ao** aorta; **az** azygos vein; **bcv** brachiocephalic vein; **cc** cricoid cartilage; **cca** common carotid artery; **cs** carotid sheath; **ec** external carotid artery; **ej** external jugular; **ic** internal carotid artery; **ijv** internal jugular vein; **it** inferior thyroid veins; **L** left recurrent laryngeal nerve; **oe** oesophagus; **p** phrenic nerve; **R** right recurrent laryngeal nerve; **sa** scalenus anterior; **sc** subclavian artery; **scm** sternocleidomastoid; **st** sympathetic trunk; **t** thyroid; **tc** thyroid cartilage; **tr** trachea.

SAQ 12: Trachea and Tracheostomy

a) **Briefly describe the anatomy of the trachea (6 marks)**

Begins as a continuation of the larynx below the cricoid cartilage (C6 level)
10–12 cm in length (half cervical, half thoracic), 2.5 cm diameter
Terminates at the plane of the sternal angle (T4/5 IV disc) at mid-inspiration (but varies with phase of respiration – more inferior in inspiration and superior in expiration)
Structure maintained by 15–20 C-shaped rings of hyaline cartilage, joined by fibro-elastic tissue
Posteriorly, trachealis (smooth muscle) joins the ends of the cartilages
Lined by pseudostratified, columnar epithelium (containing goblet cells)
Blood supply/venous drainage: inferior thyroid artery and bronchial arteries, drains to inferior thyroid veins
Nerve supply: recurrent branches of vagus nerve supply mucosa (including pain fibres), upper ganglia of sympathetic trunks supply smooth muscle and blood vessels (vasomotor)

b) **List relations of the trachea in the neck (C6) and thorax (T4) (8 marks)**

Neck:
- Anteriorly: anterior jugular veins, sternohyoid, sternothyroid, isthmus of thyroid gland (overlying second–fourth tracheal cartilages), inferior thyroid veins, thyroid ima artery
- Laterally: lobes of the thyroid gland, carotid sheath (common carotid artery, internal jugular vein, vagus nerve)
- Posteriorly: oesophagus, recurrent laryngeal nerves (in tracheo-oesophageal grove)

Thorax:
- Anteriorly: left brachycephalic vein, brachiocephalic trunk, left common carotid artery, arch of aorta, thymus
- Left: arch of aorta (**'red arch'**), left common carotid artery, left subclavian artery, left recurrent laryngeal nerve, pleura
- Right: azygos vein (**'blue arch'**), right CN 10, pleura
- Posteriorly: oesophagus, left recurrent laryngeal nerve

c) **List immediate/early and late complications of a tracheostomy placed between the second and third tracheal rings (6 marks)**

Immediate/early:
- From instrumentation: bleeding, tracheal cartilage fracture, posterior tracheal wall/oesophageal injury, pneumothorax, laryngeal nerve damage
- From loss of airway: hypoxia, false passage, surgical emphysema

Late:
- From instrumentation: bleeding, infection
- From loss of airway: hypoxia, displacement, blockage
- From scarring: tracheal stenosis, tracheo-oesophageal fistula, trachea granuloma, vocal changes, persistent stoma, dysphagia, disfiguring scar, tracheomalacia

Section 3

OSCE Stations 1–18 (Answers)

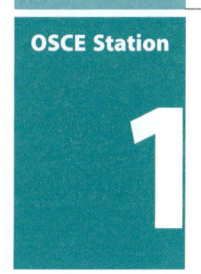

OSCE Station 1

Ankle Block

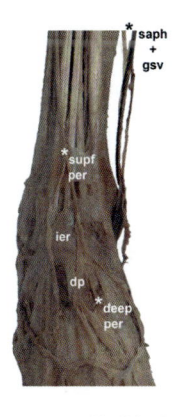

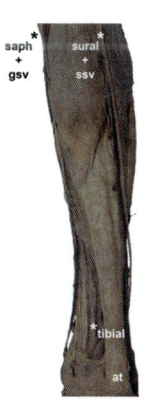

a.

b.

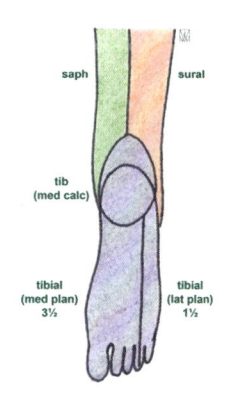

OSCE1 Ankle block. a. Dissection of dorsum of foot and posterior view of leg. b. Cutaneous nerve distribution in leg and foot. **at** Achilles tendon; **dp** dorsalis pedis artery; **gsv** great saphenous vein; **ier** inferior extensor retinaculum; **lat plan** lateral plantar; **med calc** medial calcaneal; **med plan** medial plantar; **per** peroneal; **saph** saphenous; **ssv** small saphenous vein.

a) Name the nerves labelled A–E. Describe their area of cutaneous innervation (10 marks)
   A) Tibial*
      Lies posterior to the medial malleolus, typically posterior to the posterior tibial artery**
      Gives medial calcaneal branches, which pierce flexor retinaculum to supply the skin of the heel (including weight-bearing surface)
      Divides into the medial and lateral plantar nerves in the foot (under flexor retinaculum), which provide cutaneous innervation to the sole of the foot (medial 3½ toes and lateral 1½ toes respectively)***
      Also supplies skin over distal phalanges
   B) Saphenous
      Largest sensory branch of the femoral nerve
      Below the knee it travels with the great/long saphenous vein
      Sensation to medial calf and medial aspect of the ankle/foot (as far as first MTPJ – 'bunion area')

C) Sural
   Formed by the union of branches of the tibial and common peroneal nerves
   Below the knee it travels with the small/short saphenous vein
   Passes *posterior* to the lateral malleolus (cf. saphenous nerve and GSV lie *anterior* to the medial malleolus)
   Innervation to the lateral aspect of the calf, ankle and foot (including little toe)
D) Deep peroneal/fibular
   Common peroneal divides into superficial and deep branches within peroneus longus
   Deep nerve provides sensory supply to 1st web space
E) Superficial peroneal/fibular
   Pierces deep fascia in the distal third (between middle and distal thirds) of the leg (emerges between extensor digitorum longus and peroneus brevis)
   Sensation to lower half of anterolateral leg and ankle, dorsum of the foot via medial and lateral branches

> *There is no *posterior* tibial nerve! (This terminology has been replaced, it is now simply the tibial nerve, but is still seen in clinical texts)
> **Mnemonic for the structures behind the medial malleolus (from anterior to posterior):
>
> '**T**om, **D**ick **A**nd **V**ery **N**aughty **H**arry'
>
> **T**ibialis posterior, **F**DL, posterior tibial **A**rtery and **V**ein, tibial **N**erve, F**H**L
> ***Aide-memoire for distribution of plantar nerves: medial plantar (like median nerve on palm of the hand), lateral plantar (like ulnar nerve)

b) **Identify structures F–I (4 marks)**
   F) Achilles tendon
   G) Dorsalis pedis artery
   H) (Inferior) extensor retinaculum
   I) Small/short saphenous vein

c) **Which of these nerves lie superficial to deep fascia at the level blocked? (3 marks)**
   Saphenous
   Superficial peroneal/fibular
   Sural

d) **From time of injection to onset of block, which of these nerves classically takes the longest and why? Why is it the only nerve for which a nerve stimulator would be useful? (3 marks)**
   Tibial takes the longest as it is the largest nerve
   It is the only nerve in this block with a motor component (saphenous, deep peroneal/fibular, superficial peroneal/fibular and sural are sensory branches at this level)

Section 3
OSCE Stations 1–18 (Answers)

OSCE Station 2
Base of Skull, Foramina and Extradural Haematoma

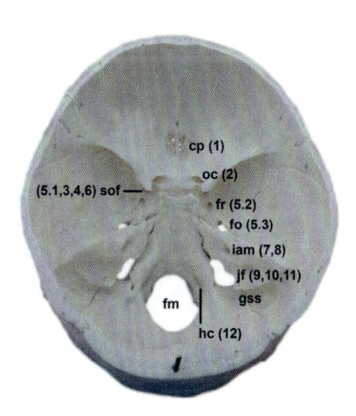

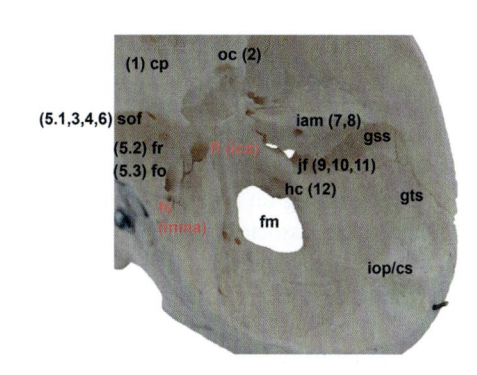

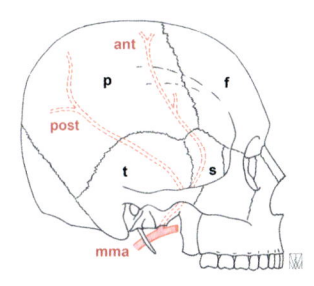

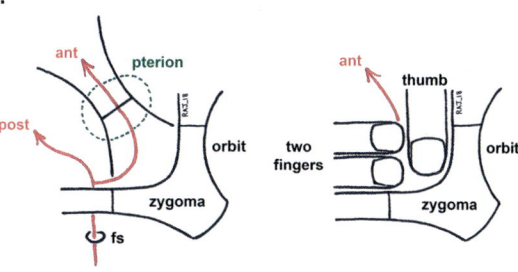

OSCE2 Base of skull. a. Foramina in base of skull. b. Pterion and middle meningeal artery. c. Surface marking of pterion. **cp** cribriform plate; **f** frontal; **fl** foramen lacerum; **fm** foramen magnum; **fo** foramen ovale; **fr** foramen rotundum; **fs** foramen spinosum; **gss** groove for sigmoid sinus; **gts** groove for transverse sinus; **hc** hypoglossal canal; **iam** internal acoustic meatus; **ica** internal carotid artery; **iop/cs** internal occipital protuberance/confluence of sinuses; **jf** jugular foramen; **mma** middle meningeal artery; **oc** optic canal; **p** parietal; **s** sphenoid; **sof** superior orbital fissure; **t** temporal.

a) From the image, name structures 1–5 and the nerves that pass through them (10 marks)
   1) Cribriform plate of ethmoid bone (CN 1)
   2) Optic canal (CN 2)
   3) Foramen rotundum (CN 5.2/maxillary division)
   4) Foramen ovale (CN 5.3/mandibular division, lesser petrosal nerve from CN 9)
   5) Internal auditory/acoustic meatus (CN 7 including nervus intermedius, CN 8)

b) **Name the landmarks labelled A–C and the venous sinus associated with them (3 marks)**
   A) Groove for transverse sinus (transverse venous sinus)
   B) Groove for sigmoid sinus (sigmoid venous sinus)
   C) Internal occipital protuberance (confluence of sinuses)

c) **On the image, demonstrate the boundaries of the anterior, middle and posterior cranial fossae. Describe the principal part and function of the brain associated with each (3 marks)**
   Anterior cranial fossa (frontal lobe): emotion/personality/behaviour, primary motor cortex
   Middle cranial fossa (temporal lobe): auditory processing, memory and language
   Posterior cranial fossa (cerebellum): coordinates and regulates voluntary movement (integrates sensory input from spinal cord to motor control for coordination and precision)

d) **What is the name of the region indicated by D? What clinical condition is associated with trauma in this territory and why? What are the clinical features? (4 marks)**
   Pterion – a region on the lateral side of the skull where the plate of bone is thin (see surface marking on illustration)
   Trauma here is associated with extradural haematoma because the anterior division of the middle meningeal artery lies on the deep surface, which can be damaged if the overlying bone is fractured
   Clinical features:
   - Initial lucid interval after trauma
   - Subsequent rising ICP with headache, vomiting, confusion, deteriorating consciousness and seizures
   - CN 3 palsy (ipsilateral dilated pupil in 'down and out' position)*
   - Contralateral homonymous hemianopia
   - Contralateral hemiparesis/brisk reflexes and subsequent features of brain herniation

*CN 3 palsy begins with a dilated ('blown') pupil and then adopts the 'down and out' position – the parasympathetic nerve fibres travel on the outside of the nerve and so are affected first by compression on the tentorium cerebelli, before the motor fibres are then compromised

Section 3 OSCE Stations 1–18 (Answers)

OSCE Station 3

Blood Supply of the Upper Limb and Allen's Test

a.

b.

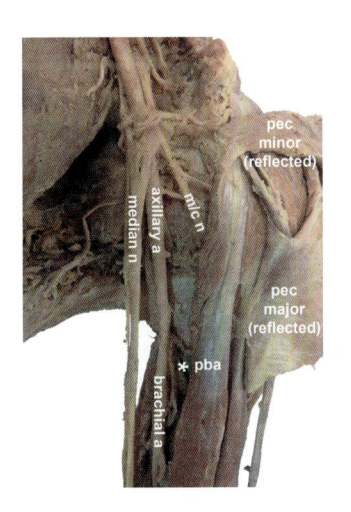

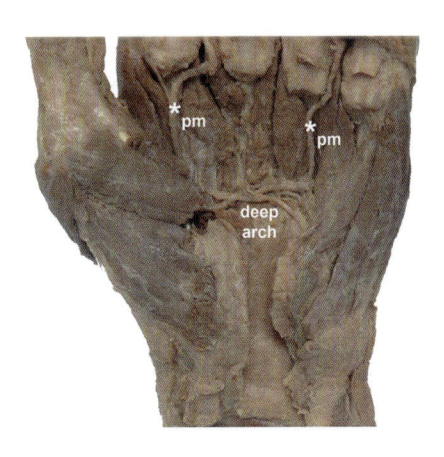

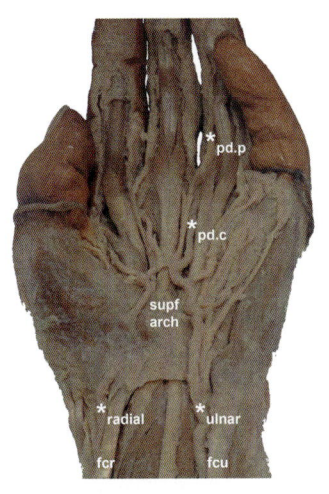

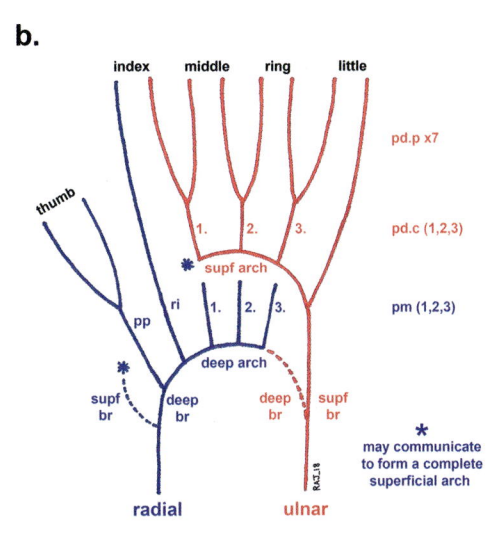

OSCE3 Blood supply of hand. a. Dissection of axilla and hand. b. Schematic of arterial supply to hand. **fcr** flexor carpi radialis; **fcu** flexor carpi ulnaris; **m/c** musculocutaneous; **pba** profunda brachii artery; **pd.c** palmar digital common (artery); **pd.p** palmar digital proper (artery); **pec** pectoralis; **pm** palmar metacarpal (artery); **pp** princeps pollicis (artery); **ri** radialis indicis (artery).

a) **Identify structures A–E in these cadaveric images (5 marks)**
   A) Axillary artery
   B) Radial artery
   C) Brachial artery
   D) Deep palmar arch
   E) Superficial palmar arch

b) **Name the artery running with the following nerve (3 marks)**
   Radial nerve in the proximal arm: profunda brachii artery
   Median nerve in the cubital fossa: brachial artery
   Ulnar nerve at the wrist: ulnar artery

c) **Describe collateral arterial supply of hand (8 marks)**
   Supplied from radial and ulnar arteries (arise from the brachial artery at the level of the neck of the radius, in the cubital fossa)
   They enter the hand to form two arterial arches: superficial (principally from the ulnar) and deep (principally from the radial)
   Radial artery:
   - Palpable at the wrist, then continues through the anatomical snuff box as the 'deep branch' to form the deep palmar arch (which is completed by the deep branch of the ulnar artery)
   - Gives a superficial branch 2 cm proximal to the wrist crease (passes over the flexor retinaculum, through the thenar muscles and contributes to the superficial arch)

   Ulnar artery:
   - Palpable at the wrist, then continues over the flexor retinaculum (in canal of Guyon) to form the superficial palmar arch (completed by the superficial branch of the radial artery)
   - Gives a deep branch (through the hypothenar muscles), which contributes to the deep arch

   Palmar arches:
   - Superficial: supplies medial 3½ digits via palmar digital arteries (cf. opposite to the ulnar nerve distribution, which provides sensory supply to the medial 1½ digits)
   - Deep: supplies the lateral 1½ digits via princeps policis and radialis indicis arteries (cf. median nerve provides sensory supply to the lateral 3½ digits)
   - The two arches are also linked by metacarpal arteries

d) **What is Allen's test? (4 marks)**
   Used before attempting cannulation of the radial artery
   Test to assess adequate ulnar collateral supply to the hand
   Compress radial and ulnar arteries at the wrist
   Elevate hand and make a fist for 30 seconds
   When opening the hand and the hand is pale (due to limited arterial supply)
   Release the ulnar artery: colour should return to the hand within 10 seconds
   Poor ulnar arterial supply is indicated if this is prolonged
   (The accuracy of this test is questioned)

Section 3: OSCE Stations 1–18 (Answers)

OSCE Station 4: Brachial Plexus and Supra/Infraclavicular Blocks

OSCE4 Brachial plexus. a. Dissection of brachial plexus. b. Schematic of brachial plexus (basic pattern, above; with branches added, below). **ax** axillary; **ds** dorsal scapular; **lc** lateral cord; **lp** lateral pectoral; **lrm** lateral root of median; **lss** lower subscapular; **lt** lower trunk; **lt** long thoracic; **m** median; **mcn** musculocutaneous; **mc** medial cord; **mca** medial cutaneous nerve of arm; **mcfa** medial cutaneous nerve of forearm; **mp** medial pectoral; **mrm** medial root of median; **mt** middle trunk; **ns** nerve to subclavius; **rad** radial; **ss** suprascapular; **td** thoracodorsal; **u** ulnar; **uss** upper subscapular; **ut** upper trunk.

a) Name structures A–E on this image of the brachial plexus (5 marks)
   A) C6 nerve root
   B) Superior trunk
   C) Lateral cord
   D) Lateral pectoral nerve
   E) Medial cutaneous nerve of the arm

b) **Name the nerve roots that contribute to the nerves labelled F–I (4 marks)**
   F) Ulnar nerve: C8–T1 (sometimes C7)
   G) Radial nerve: C5–T1
   H) Median nerve: C5–T1
   I) Axillary nerve: C5–6
c) **What motor response is demonstrated on stimulation of the lateral, posterior and medial cords of the brachial plexus? (3 marks)**
   Posterior cord: wrist/finger extension
   Medial cord: thumb adduction, wrist flexion
   Lateral cord: elbow flexion, forearm supination
d) **Name the part(s) of the brachial plexus targeted by the following blocks: (4 marks)**
   Interscalene: roots
   Supraclavicular: distal trunks/proximal divisions
   Infraclavicular: cords
   Axillary: branches (peripheral nerves)
e) **What are the benefits of ultrasound-guided (over anatomical landmark or nerve stimulator) brachial plexus blocks? (4 marks)**
   Allows continuous visualisation of needle tip/placement and local anaesthetic spread
   Quicker procedure
   Faster onset
   Longer duration
   Higher success rate
   Reduced local anaesthetic volume used
   Avoidance of discomfort of nerve stimulation (especially if supplying an injury/fractured limb)
   Allows for anatomical variation and differing needle approach
   Reduced incidence of intravascular injection
   Reduced incidence of pneumothorax
   (No difference in incidence of nerve injury demonstrated in current evidence)

Section 3: OSCE Stations 1–18 (Answers)

OSCE Station 5: Circle of Willis

OSCE5 Circle of Willis. a. Schematic of circle of Willis and effects of cerebral arterial occlusion. b. Plaster model. **aca** anterior cerebral artery; **aco** anterior communicating artery; **aica** anterior inferior cerebellar artery; **as** anterior spinal; **B** Broca's area; **b** basilar; **ic** internal carotid artery; **ica** internal carotid artery; **mca** middle cerebral artery; **oc** optic chiasma; **pca** posterior cerebral artery; **pco** posterior communicating artery; **pica** posterior inferior cerebellar artery; **pit** pituitary stalk; **ps** posterior spinal; **sca** superior cerebellar artery; **v** vertebral; **W** Wernicke's area.

a) On the image OSCE5, name structures A–E (5 marks)
   A) Vertebral artery
   B) Basilar artery
   C) Posterior communicating artery
   D) Anterior cerebral artery
   E) Internal carotid artery

b) What is the origin of A and E? (2 marks)
   A) Subclavian artery (first branch of the first part)
   E) Common carotid artery (level with the superior border of thyroid cartilage – at C4)*

*Note that the common carotid artery arises from the brachiocephalic trunk on the right, and directly from the arch of the aorta on the left

c) **Where are the common locations of intracranial vascular aneurysms and with what frequencies do they occur? (6 marks)**
   Anterior communicating (40%)
   Posterior communicating (30%)
   Middle cerebral artery (20%)

d) **What is the significance of the circle of Willis? (1 mark)**
   Provides collateral circulation for the brain, compensating for reduced flow through individual segments of the arterial circle and thus maintaining blood supply to the brain

e) **Describe the speech deficit that occurs from occlusion of the:**
   i) dominant hemisphere middle cerebral artery anterior branch
   ii) dominant hemisphere middle cerebral artery posterior branch
   iii) dominant hemisphere middle cerebral artery (3 marks)

   i) expressive dysphasia (anterior speech area of Broca)
   ii) receptive dysphasia (posterior speech area of Wernicke)
   iii) global aphasia

f) **Which artery has been affected in a patient suffering from an occlusive stroke presenting with:**
   i) motor/sensory deficit of the contralateral lower limb
   ii) contralateral homonymous hemianopia with macular sparing
   iii) motor/sensory deficit of the contralateral upper limb and face (3 marks)

   i) ACA
   ii) PCA**
   iii) MCA

**Note that the MCA often supplies the macular part of the visual area, hence sparing

Section 3
OSCE Stations 1–18 (Answers)

OSCE Station 6
Vagus Nerve

a.

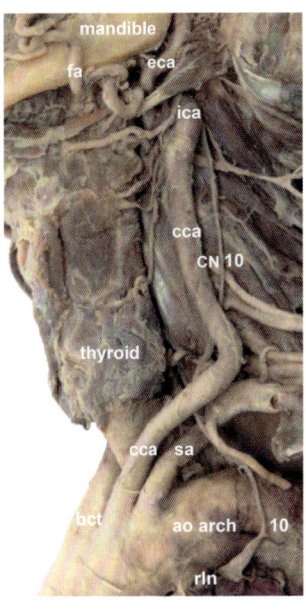

b.

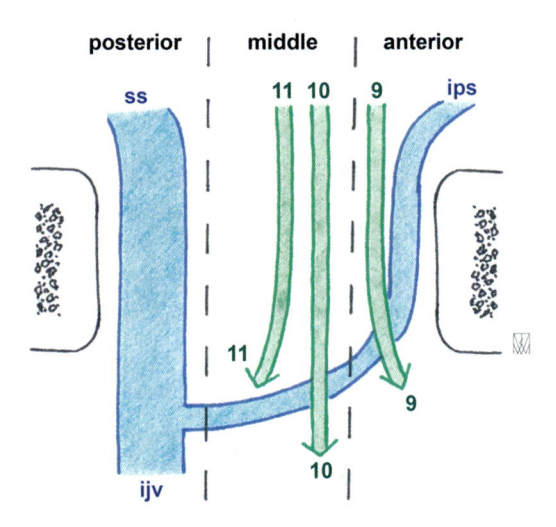

OSCE6 Vagus nerve. a. Dissection of left side of neck and superior mediastinum. b. Jugular foramen and compartments/contents. **CN 10** vagus nerve; **ao** aorta; **bct** brachiocephalic trunk; **cca** common carotid artery; **eca** external carotid artery; **fa** facial artery; **ica** internal carotid artery; **ijv** internal jugular vein; **ips** inferior petrosal sinus; **rln** recurrent laryngeal nerve; **sa** subclavian artery; **ss** sigmoid sinus.

a) **Name the nerve labelled A on the image OSCE6 (1 mark)**
   CN 10 (vagus nerve)

b) **From which nuclei does it arise? (4 marks)**
   Dorsal nucleus of vagus (parasympathetic: heart, lungs, gut)
   Nucleus ambiguus (motor: skeletal muscle of palate, larynx, pharynx)
   Nucleus of tractus solitarius (special sense: taste from epiglottis, cardiorespiratory and vomiting reflexes)
   Sensory nuclei of trigeminal (general sense: larynx/pharynx, dura of posterior cranial fossa, ear*)

*CN 10 supply to ear: lower half of outer surface of tympanic membrane, external auditory meatus and small area behind auricle

c) **What is the name of this foramen (B) in the base of the skull? (1 mark)**
   Jugular foramen
d) **Which structures pass through it? (4 marks)**
   Anterior compartment:
   - Inferior petrosal sinus
   - CN 9

   Middle compartment:
   - CN 10 and 11

   Posterior compartment:
   - Sigmoid sinus (becoming continuous with IJV)
e) **What is structure C (a branch of A)? To which vascular structure is it most closely related on the left and on the right? (4 marks)**
   Left recurrent laryngeal nerve
   - Left: arch of aorta
   - Right: subclavian artery
f) **What stimuli can increase the outflow of the nerve labelled A, and what effects are seen during anaesthesia? (6 marks)**
   Effects:
   - Bradycardia, asystole in severe circumstances
   - Laryngospasm (Brewer–Luckhardt reflex: laryngospasm provoked by distant stimuli)
   - Bronchospasm

   Stimuli:
   - Dura (e.g. subarachnoid haemorrhage)
   - Zygoma (e.g. surgery, trauma)
   - Extraocular muscles, particularly medial rectus (e.g. eye surgery)
   - Carotid sinus (e.g. carotid sinus massage)
   - Pharynx and glottis (e.g. intubation of child when hooking epiglottis)
   - Bronchial tree
   - Heart
   - Mesentery and peritoneum (e.g. insufflation during laparoscopy)
   - Bladder and urethra
   - Testis, uterus and cervix (e.g. exteriorising uterus, gynaecological surgery, PV bleed)
   - Rectum and anus (e.g. anal stretch)

Section 3
OSCE Stations 1–18 (Answers)

OSCE Station 7
Coronary Circulation

a.

sternocostal surface (view from front)

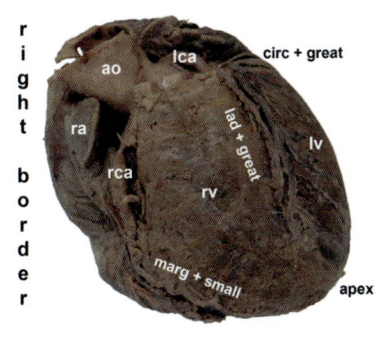

diaphragmatic surface (view from below)

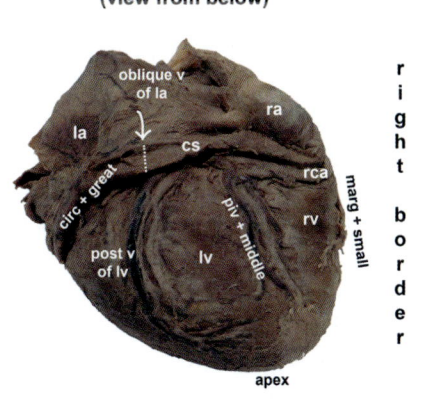

heart & right border flipped in this direction

b.

c. fetal position — adult position

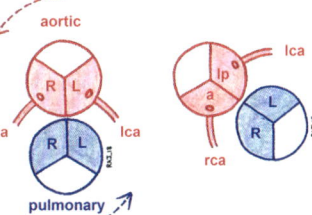

OSCE7 Heart. a. Dissection. b. Schematic of coronary vessels. c. Schematic to explain the nomenclature of the aortic valve cusps in the fetus and adult. **a** anterior; **ac** anterior cardiac veins; **ao** aorta; **av** AV nodal artery; **circ** circumflex artery; **cs** coronary sinus; **great** great cardiac vein; **la** left atrium; **lad** left anterior descending artery; **lca** left coronary artery; **lp** left posterior; **lv** left ventricle; **marg** marginal artery; **middle** middle cardiac vein; **piv** posterior interventricular artery; **post v** posterior vein; **ra** right atrium; **rca** right coronary artery; **rv** right ventricle; **sa** SA nodal artery; **small** small cardiac vein; **vcm** venae cordis minimae.

Section 3: OSCE Stations 1–18 (Answers)

a) **Name structures A–D on these images of the heart (4 marks)**
  A) Left coronary artery
  B) Anterior interventricular/left anterior descending artery
  C) Right (acute) marginal artery
  D) Posterior interventricular/descending artery

b) **Name structures E–H (4 marks)**
  E) Coronary sinus
  F) Great cardiac vein
  G) Middle cardiac vein
  H) Small cardiac vein

c) **From where do the main coronary arteries arise? (2 marks)**
  RCA: right* (anterior**) aortic sinus (of ascending aorta)
  LCA: left* (left posterior**) aortic sinus (of ascending aorta)

> Nomeclature relating to the coronary sinuses:
> - *Fetal position: right (RCA), left (LCA), posterior (non-coronary)
> - **Adult position: anterior (RCA), right posterior (non-coronary), left posterior (LCA)
>
> The fetal terminology is typically used in clinical practice

d) **What proportion of the cardiac output is supplied to the myocardium? (1 mark)**
  5% or 250 ml/minute (can increase fivefold during exercise)

e) **What is meant by coronary arterial dominance? (1 mark)**
  This is defined by the vessel that gives rise to the posterior interventricular artery (usually RCA), as this in turn gives rise to the AV nodal artery

f) **Which artery supplies the AV node and where does it arise from? (2 marks)**
  AV nodal artery
  In >80% it is from the RCA, in 10% it is a continuation of the circumflex branch of the LCA
  <10% have a 'balanced' circulation where the AV node is supplied by both the RCA and circumflex (LCA): branches of both sides run in or near the posterior interventricular groove

g) **Which artery supplies the SA node and where does it arise from? (2 marks)**
  SA nodal artery
  In 60% it arises from the RCA, in 40% from the circumflex artery (LCA)

h) **What are the ECG features of right coronary artery occlusion? (2 marks)**
  Inferior MI: features in leads II, III and aVF
  ST segmental elevation (subsequent development of Q waves)
  (Reciprocal ST depression in aVL +/− V1)
  Other features: heart block, right bundle branch block

i) **Describe the difference between a type I and type II acute myocardial infarction? (2 marks)**

A type I MI describes focal myocardial ischaemia/necrosis resulting from a lesion in specific coronary artery (most commonly rupture of an atheromatous plaque)

A type II MI describes myocardial ischaemia/necrosis from an oxygen supply/demand mismatch (e.g. secondary to fast atrial fibrillation/severe tachycardia and hypotension), a coronary abnormality may not be present

Section 3: OSCE Stations 1–18 (Answers)

OSCE Station 8: Diaphragm

a.

b.

OSCE8 Diaphragm. a. and b. Structures passing through the diaphragm and major vertebral levels. **ao** aorta; **az** azygos vein; **cc** cisterna chyli; **haz** hemiazygos vein; **ivc** inferior vena cava; **L gast** left gastric vessels; **oe** oesophagus; **phren** phrenic; **pm** psoas major; **ql** quadratus lumborum; **sp** splanchnic nerves; **st** sympathetic trunk; **sup epi** superior epigastric vessels; **td** thoracic duct; **vta** vagal trunk (anterior); **vtp** vagal trunk (posterior).

a) On the diagram OSCE8, name structures A, B and C. State at what vertebral level they pass through the diaphragm, and name a structure they travel with at this level (9 marks)
   A) Inferior vena cava
      - Vena caval opening: T8
      - Transmits: IVC, right phrenic nerve
   B) Oesophagus
      - Oesophageal opening: T10
      - Transmits: oesophagus, vagal trunks (anterior and posterior), left gastric vessels, lymphatics from lower third of oesophagus
   C) Aorta (junction of descending thoracic aorta/abdominal aorta)
      - Aortic hiatus: T12
      - Transmits: aorta, azygos vein (on right of aorta) and thoracic duct (between them)

OSCE Station 8: Diaphragm

Easy to remember!
- Vena cava – 8 letters
- Oesophagus – 10 letters
- Aortic hiatus – 12 letters

b) **What is structure D, and what is it derived from? (1 mark)**
D) Central tendon* (derived from the septum transversum)

*Sometimes referred to as a *trefoil* tendon because it has three rounded lobes

c) **At which point does the left phrenic nerve pierce the diaphragm? (1 mark)**
Apex beat of the heart (5th ICS on the left, in the midclavicular line)

d) **Describe the nerve supply of the diaphragm (3 marks)**
Motor supply: phrenic nerves only (C3/4/5**)
Sensory supply:
- Central part: phrenic nerve (C3/4/5)
- Peripheral part: lower six intercostal/thoracoabdominal nerves (T7–12)

**C3/4/5 keep the diaphragm alive!

e) **What is the normal level of the diaphragm in the midclavicular line? (2 marks)**
Left hemidiaphragm: 5th intercostal space
Right hemidiaphragm: 5th rib
N.B. These are values for mid-inspiration, therefore lower on CXR as taken during inspiration

f) **What are the potential causes of a raised unilateral or bilateral hemidiaphragm? (4 marks)**
Unilateral:
- Phrenic nerve palsy
- Lobar/lung collapse

Bilateral:
- Poor inspiratory effort
- Restrictive lung disease
- Gastrointestinal obstruction/ileus
- Ascites
- Pregnancy
- Obesity
- Other (e.g. intra-abdominal mass)

Section 3

OSCE Stations 1–18 (Answers)

OSCE Station 9

Dural Venous Sinuses and Cavernous Sinus Thrombosis

a.

b.

c.

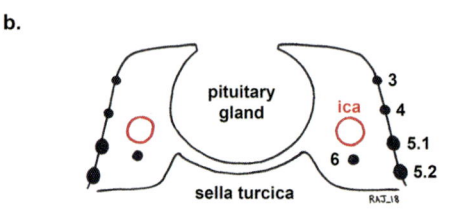

OSCE9 Dural venous sinuses. a. Dural venous sinuses. b. Schematic coronal section through cavernous sinus. c. Schematic to explain the effects of cavernous sinus thrombosis following infection in the danger area of the face. **cs** cavernous sinus; **fo** foramen ovale; **gc** great cerebral vein; **ica** internal carotid artery; **ijv** internal jugular vein; **inf pet s** inferior petrosal sinus; **ips** inferior petrosal sinus; **iss** inferior sagittal sinus; **pp** pterygoid plexus; **sis** sigmoid sinus; **sov** superior ophthalmic veins; **sphs** sphenoparietal sinus; **sps** superior petrosal sinus; **sss** superior sagittal sinus; **sts** straight sinus; **sup oph** superior ophthalmic veins; **supf mid cerebral** superficial middle cerebral vein; **ts** transverse sinus.

a) **Name structures A–E on the image OSCE9 (5 marks)**
   A) Superior sagittal sinus
   B) Inferior sagittal sinus
   C) Straight sinus
   D) Left transverse sinus
   E) Right sigmoid sinus

b) **What drains to and from structure F? (5 marks)**
   Structure F: cavernous sinus
   Receives: ophthalmic veins (superior and inferior), cerebral veins (superficial middle cerebral +/− inferior cerebral), sphenoparietal sinus
   Drains to: petrosal sinuses (superior and inferior)
   N.B. The intercavernous sinuses (anterior and posterior) communicate between the two cavernous sinuses, and emissary veins connect the cavernous sinus and pterygoid venous plexus below

c) **What structures lie within structure F? (5 marks)**

Within the sinus:
- Internal carotid artery (carrying postganglionic sympathetic fibres of the internal carotid plexus, including those for dilator pupillae and levator palpebrae superioris)
- CN 6
- (Venous blood)

In the lateral wall:
- CN 3
- CN 4
- CN 5.1 and 5.2

d) **What are the clinical features of thrombosis of structure F? (5 marks)**

Features of raised ICP:
- Symptoms: headache, nausea/vomiting, falling level of consciousness, seizures
- Signs: papilloedema, dropping GCS, CN 3/6 palsy

Features related to the cavernous sinus anatomy:
- CN 3–6 palsies
- Impaired venous drainage of the eye (proptosis, chemosis and injected eye)

Section 3: OSCE Stations 1–18 (Answers)

OSCE Station 10: Inguinal Regional and Hernia

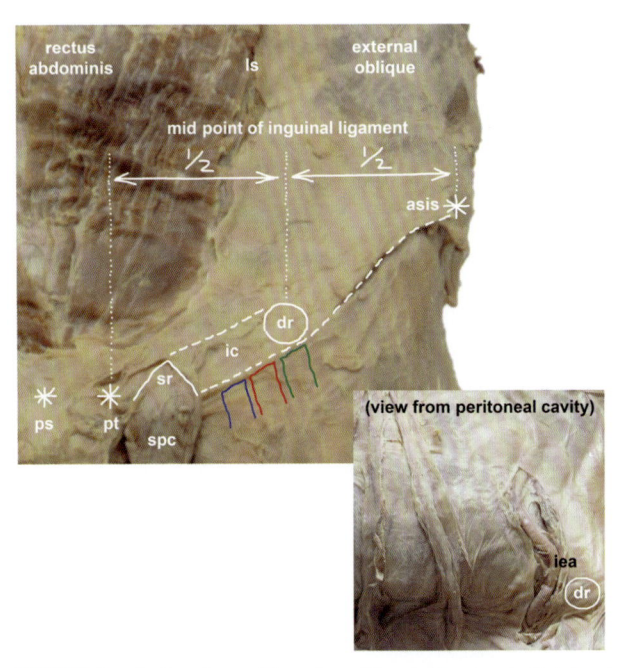

a.

b.

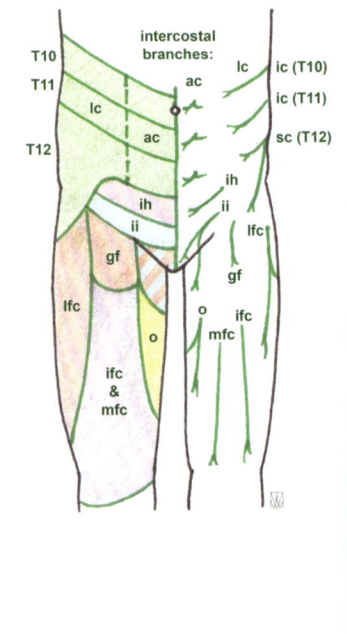

OSCE10 Inguinal region. a. Dissection of inguinal region. b. Peripheral nerve distribution in lower trunk and thighs. **ac** anterior cutaneous; **asis** anterior superior iliac spine; **dr** deep ring; **gf** genitofemoral (femoral branch); **ic** inguinal canal; **iea** inferior epigastric artery; **ifc** intermediate femoral cutaneous; **ih** iliohypogastric; **ii** ilioinguinal; **lc** lateral cutaneous; **lfc** lateral femoral cutaneous; **ls** linea semilunaris; **mfc** medial femoral cutaneous; **o** obturator; **ps** pubic symphysis; **pt** pubic tubercle; **sc** subcostal; **spc** spermatic cord; **sr** superficial ring.

a) Name structures A–F on this image (6 marks)
 A) Spermatic cord
 B) Superficial inguinal ring
 C) Deep inguinal ring
 D) Pubic tubercle
 E) Anterior superior iliac spine
 F) Inferior epigastric artery

OSCE Station 10: Inguinal Regional and Hernia

b) **On the diagram, identify the areas supplied by the nerves numbered 1–5 (5 marks)**
   1) Lateral cutaneous branch of intercostal nerve T10
   2) Iliohypogastric nerve (T12 and L1)
   3) Ilioinguinal nerve (L1)
   4) Genitofemoral nerve (femoral branch; L1–2)
   5) Lateral cutaneous nerve of thigh (L2–3)

c) **What methods of anaesthesia may be employed for inguinal hernia repair? (3 marks)**
   General anaesthesia
   Spinal anaesthesia (or epidural)
   Local anaesthesia:
   - Local infiltration
   - Iliohypogastric/ilioinguinal nerve block
   - TAP block
   - Caudal block

d) **Describe how you would manage a patient who was having inguinal hernia repair under local anaesthesia infiltration and was beginning to experience discomfort (6 marks)**
   Ask the surgeon to stop
   Speak to the patient:
   - Offer reassurance
   - Confirm the nature of the discomfort (some sort of sensation is expected)
   - If pain, determine the level of discomfort (mild/moderate/severe)

   Mild pain:
   - Further local anaesthesia infiltration
   - Intravenous opiate analgesia (e.g. fentanyl)
   - Nitrous oxide or intravenous remifentanil/propofol sedation/analgesia

   Severe pain:
   - Confirm with the surgeon the extent of surgery undertaken/still to perform
   - With a significant proportion of the operation still to perform, consider alternative/ additional technique: TAP/nerve block (if the maximal dose of local anaesthetic permits) or spinal/GA (depending on patient suitability and concern over sterility/ repositioning)

   Postoperatively:
   - Debrief patient and offer apology as appropriate

Section 3
OSCE Stations 1–18 (Answers)

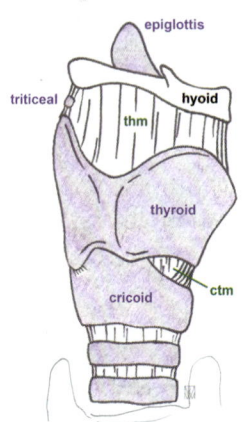

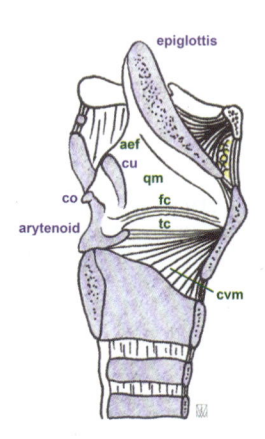

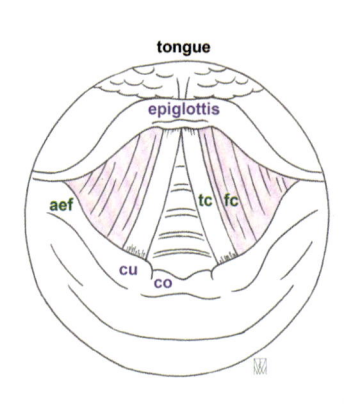

OSCE Station 11
Larynx

OSCE11 Larynx. a. Laryngeal cartilages and membranes. b. Intubation view of larynx. **aef** aryepiglottic fold; **co** corniculate cartilage; **ctm** cricothyroid membrane; **cu** cuneiform cartilage; **cvm** cricovocal membrane; **fc** false vocal cord; **qm** quadrangular membrane; **tc** true vocal cord; **thm** thyrohyoid membrane.

a) Name structures A–D on the diagram OSCE11 (4 marks)
   A) Epiglottis (elastic cartilage)
   B) Thyroid cartilage (hyaline cartilage)
   C) Cricoid cartilage (hyaline cartilage)
   D) Arytenoid cartilages (hyaline cartilage)

b) Names structures E–I (5 marks)
   E) Thyrohyoid membrane
   F) Cricothyroid membrane
   G) Aryepiglottic fold
   H) Vestibular fold (false cords)
   I) Cricovocal membrane (upper edges form the true vocal cords)

c) Describe the innervation of the larynx (3 marks)
   Superior laryngeal nerve:
   - Internal branch (sensation above vocal cords: from dorsum of epiglottis to cords)
   - External branch* (motor supply to cricothyroid)

Recurrent laryngeal nerve:
- Sensation below the vocal cords
- Motor supply to all intrinsic muscles of the larynx except cricothyroid

*Occasionally also supplies the cricopharyngeus part of the interior constrictor of the pharynx

d) **How might injury to the vagus nerve or its branches affect the larynx? (4 marks)**
Superior laryngeal nerve**: reduced vocal cord tension, hoarse voice
Recurrent laryngeal nerve:
- Complete lesion: ipsilateral vocal cord adopts a position midway between abduction/adduction
- Partial lesion***: ipsilateral vocal cord adopts a midline/adducted position (because adductors are stronger than abductors)

**Reduced sensation in the upper larynx also poses an aspiration risk
***Bilateral partial lesions lead to **complete airway obstruction** as both cords adopt the midline position (Semon's law)

e) **How can you anaesthetise the larynx for an awake fibre-optic intubation? (4 marks)**
Nebulised lignocaine
Topical local anaesthetic using a mucosal atomiser device (nasal mucosa, naso-/oro-/laryngopharynx)
'Spray as you go' (laryngopharynx, larynx, trachea)
Translaryngeal approach**** (cricothyroid puncture) is sometimes used
Nerve blocks: anterior glossopharyngeal, superior thyroid (rarely used)
Cocaine-soaked pledgets (again, rarely used)
Coadministration of sedation can reduce local anaesthetic requirement (e.g. TCI propofol or remifentanil)

****Introduces local anaesthetic to the lower airway by inserting a needle through the cricothyroid membrane and injecting – asking the patient to take a deep breath takes the local anaesthetic into the lower airway and often precipitates coughing, which further disperses the anaesthetic around the upper airway

Section 3 — OSCE Stations 1–18 (Answers)

OSCE Station 12: The Liver and Portal Venous System

a) **Name structures A–E on the image OSCE12 (5 marks)**
   A) Left lobe of the liver
   B) Gall bladder
   C) Groove for inferior vena cava
   D) Ligamentum teres (or round ligament of liver; obliterated (left) umbilical vein that lies in the free edge of the falciform ligament)
   E) Fissure for ligamentum venosum

b) **Describe the microscopic architecture of the liver (6 marks)**

   Numerous ways to describe this, based around the portal triad, a hepatic lobule or acinus

   Portal triads run throughout the liver, which consist of:
   - Arteriole (branch of hepatic artery proper)
   - Venule (branch of the hepatic portal vein)
   - Bile ductule (tributary of the biliary tree/bile duct)
   - (And other structures, e.g. lymphatic vessels)

   Around these lie hepatic lobules:
   - Columnar structure
   - In cross-section is hexagonal in shape and around 1 mm in diameter
   - Consists of hepatocytes layered around a central venule (which drains to hepatic vein and then the inferior vena cava)
   - The edges abut other lobules, the corners converge on a portal triad

   The portal triad supplies blood from the gastrointestinal tract, for the processing of absorbed enteric content

   Functionally, three zones of metabolic activity are described, centring on the portal triad:
   - Zone 1: cells closest to the perimeter of the triad, most metabolically active (greatest availability of oxygen supply from the arterial blood)
   - Zone 2: intermediate zone
   - Zone 3: least metabolically active, lowest oxygen supply (therefore vulnerable to ischaemia)

   Metabolic activity of zones are adapted to their oxygen supply (e.g. β-oxidation of fatty acids in zone 1, glycolysis in zone 3)

   Zone 3 is most susceptible to ischaemic liver injury

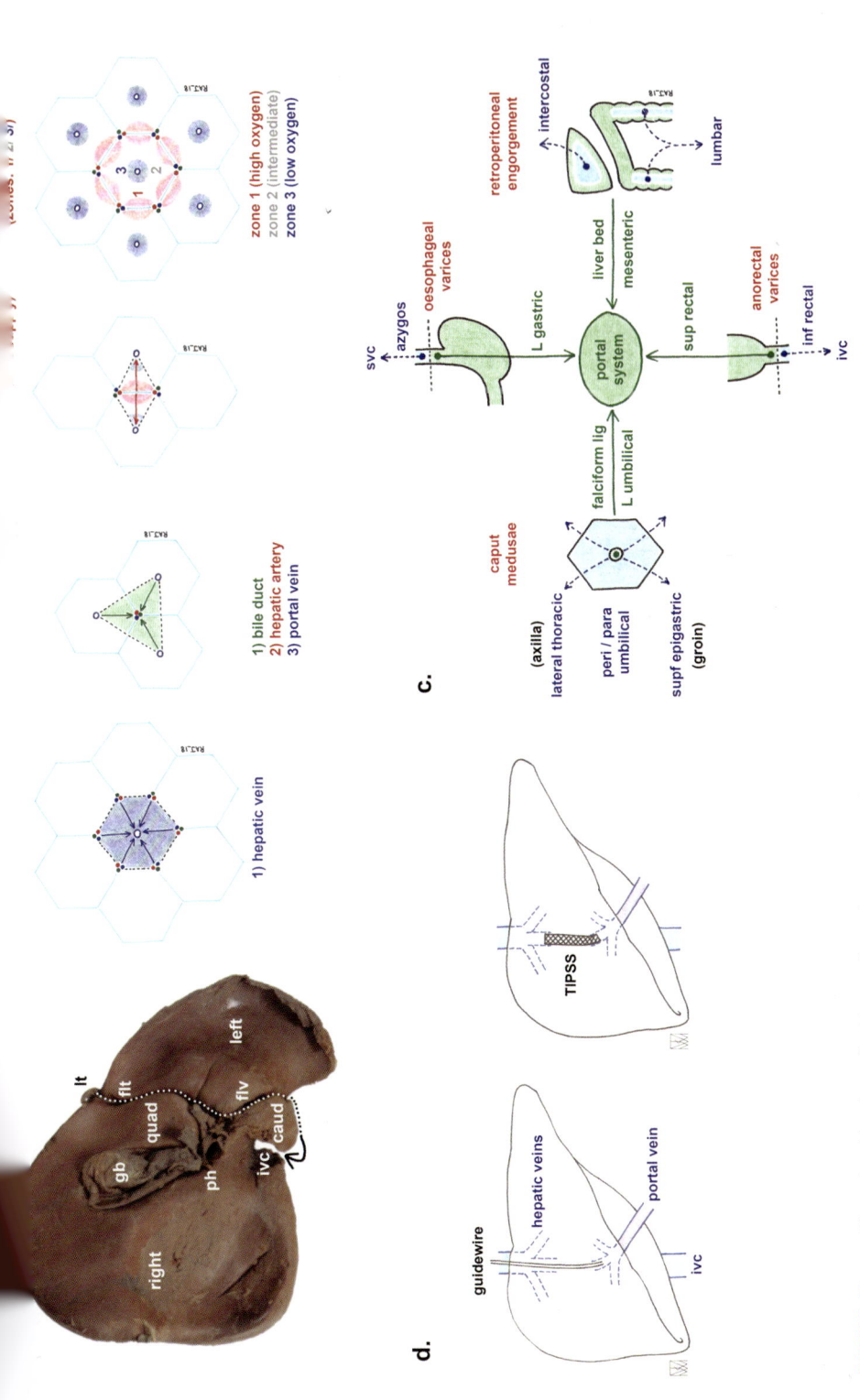

OSCE12 Liver. a. Dissection. Line shows fetal bypass from placenta to IVC. b. Histological architecture of liver (structural cf. functional). c. Sites of portosystemic anastomosis and effects of portal hypertension. d. TIPSS procedure. **caud** caudate lobe; **flt** fissure for the ligamentum teres; **flv** fissure for the ligamentum venosum; **gb** gall bladder; **ivc** inferior vena cava; **lt** ligamentum teres; **ph** porta hepatis; **quad** quadrate lobe; **svc** superior vena cava; **TIPSS** transjugular intrahepatic portosystemic shunt.

c) **Name four sites of portosystemic anastomosis (4 marks)**
   1) Lower oesophagus (connecting *left gastric vein*, draining lower third of oesophagus, with the *azygos vein*, draining middle third)
   2) Retroperitoneal veins (drain *retroperitoneal surfaces of organs* to the *body wall veins*)
   3) Bare area of the liver (drains retroperitoneal surface *liver* to *body wall veins*)
   4) Periumbilical veins (the ligamentum teres (umbilical vein) can recanalise in portal hypertension, connecting the *portal vein* with the *superior/inferior epigastric veins and anterior abdominal wall veins*)
   5) Upper anal canal (connects the *superior rectal vein* (which becomes the *inferior mesenteric vein*, draining the mid- and hindgut) with the *middle and inferior rectal veins* (which drain to the *inferior pudendal vein* and then to the *internal iliac vein*))
   6) Ductus venosus (can recanalise in portal hypertension, connecting left branch of the *portal vein* with the *inferior vena cava*)

   1) Oesophageal varices
   2) Retroperitoneal engorgement complicating surgery
   3) Same as above
   4) Caput medusae
   5) Anorectal varices
   6) Hepatic encephalopathy as portal blood with absorbed enteric products bypasses liver to systemic circulation

d) **Name the two vessels connected by a transjugular intrahepatic portosystemic shunt (TIPSS) procedure. How does this help to treat patients with liver cirrhosis? (5 marks)**
   Portal vein and hepatic vein
   In liver cirrhosis, the hepatic scarring causes constriction of the portal venous system, increasing resistance to flow
   Portal hypertension then develops causing the creation of a collateral circulation (portosystemic anastomoses – see above), which is prone to bleeding
   A TIPSS bypasses the liver, so portal blood drains directly to the systemic veins (reducing pressure in the portal system and therefore the risk/extent of bleeding)

Section 3
OSCE Stations 1–18 (Answers)

OSCE Station 13
Nose and Paranasal Air Sinuses

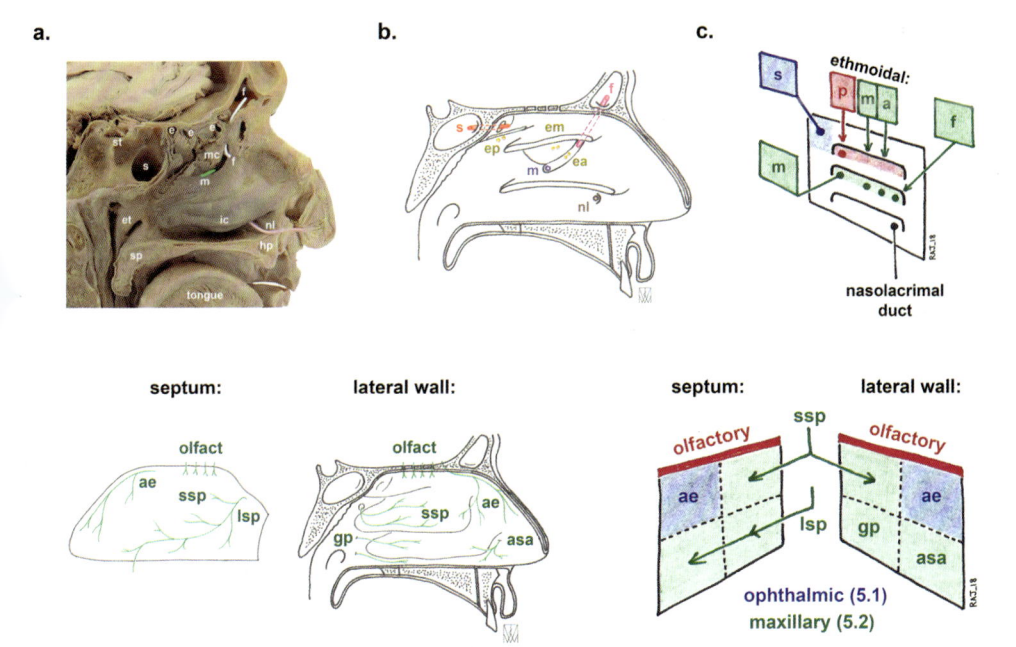

a. b. c.

OSCE13 Nose and paranasal air sinuses. a. Median section through nasal cavity. b & c. Schematics of the lateral wall of the nasal cavity and air sinus openings. Below: schematics of nerve supply of walls of nasal cavity. **ae** anterior ethmoidal nerve; **asa** anterior superior alveolar nerve; **e** Ethmoidal sinuses; **ea** ethmoidal sinus (anterior); **em** ethmoidal sinus (middle); **ep** ethmoidal sinus (posterior); **et** Eustachian tube; **f** frontal sinus; **gp** greater palatine nerve; **hp** hard palate; **ic** inferior concha; **lsp** long sphenopalatine nerve (nasopalatine nerve); **m** maxillary sinus; **mc** middle concha; **nl** nasolacrimal duct; **olfact** olfactory; **s** sphenoidal sinus; **sp** soft palate; **ssp** short sphenopalatine nerves (med & lat post sup nasal nerves); **st** sella turcica.

a) Name structures 1-10 on this image of the lateral wall of the nasal cavity (10 marks)
   1) Middle turbinate/concha (of ethmoid bone)
   2) Opening of frontal sinus
   3) Opening of maxillary sinus
   4) Opening of nasolacrimal duct
   5) Hard palate
   6) Soft palate
   7) Eustachian tube
   8) Sphenoidal air sinus
   9) Frontal air sinus
   10) Tongue

b) **Name the parent nerve from which the nerves labelled in the diagram arise (5 marks)**
Anterior ethmoidal nerve (nasal branches): continuation of nasociliary branch of ophthalmic division CN 5.1
Anterior superior alveolar nerve (nasal branches): maxillary division CN 5.2
Nasopalatine nerve: maxillary division CN 5.2
Greater and lesser palatine nerves: maxillary division CN 5.2
Olfactory nerves: CN 1

c) **List the structures/cavities passed through, before reaching the trachea, with the fibre-optic scope when performing a nasal intubation (5 marks)**
Anterior nares (nostrils)
Nasal cavity
Posterior nares (choana)
Nasopharynx
Oropharynx
Laryngopharynx
Larynx

Section 3: OSCE Stations 1–18 (Answers)

OSCE Station 14

Paravertebral Space and Block

a.

b.

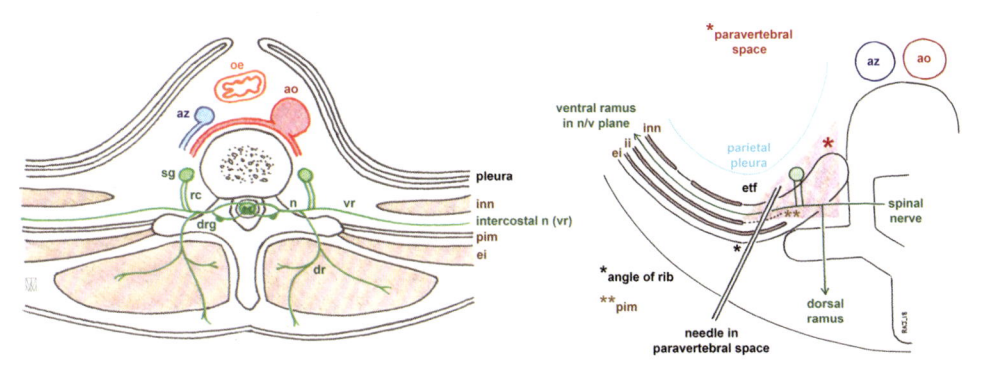

OSCE14 Paravertebral space. a. and b. Schematic of paravertebral space without and with rib. **ao** aorta; **az** azygos vein; **dr** dorsal ramus; **drg** dorsal root ganglion; **ei** external intercostals; **etf** endothoracic fascia; **ii** internal intercostals; **inn** innermost intercostals; **n** spinal nerve; **n/v** neurovascular plane; **oe** oesophagus; **pim** posterior intercostal membrane; **rc** rami communicantes; **sg** sympathetic ganglion; **vr** ventral ramus.

a) **Name structures A–E on this diagram of the paravertebral space (5 marks)**
   A) Dorsal ramus of spinal nerve
   B) Posterior intercostal membrane (from internal intercostal muscle)
   C) External intercostal muscle
   D) Parietal pleura
   E) Transverse process of vertebra

b) **Name the contents of the paravertebral space (5 marks)**
   Spinal nerve (ventral/dorsal rami)
   Intercostal artery
   Intercostal vein
   Rami communicantes of sympathetic chain with spinal nerves (white/grey)
   Paravertebral sympathetic chain
   Lymphatics
   Fat

c) **Name four complications of paravertebral block (4 marks)**
   Nerve injury
   Bilateral block (spread to the contralateral side via the epidural space)
   Epidural spread
   Intrathecal injection

Hypotension
Horner's syndrome
Pneumothorax/lung injury (in thoracic region)
Damage to abdominal retroperitoneal viscera, e.g. liver, kidney (in lumbar region)
Vascular puncture: intravascular injection and local anaesthetic systemic toxicity, bleeding

d) **Describe a technique for performing a paravertebral block (6 marks)**
Consent
Stop before you block: confirm side and site
SLIMRAG:

- Sterile procedure (wash hands, sterile gloves, sterile dressing pack)
- Light source/ultrasound
- IV access
- Monitoring (AAGBI minimum standard)
- Resuscitation drugs/equipment available
- Assistant (who is happy to assist with regional or general anaesthetic)
- General anaesthetic (ensure equipment/drugs available to convert if required)

Position: either lying on side or sitting
Clean the skin with 0.5% chlorhexidine (allow to dry)
High-frequency linear/curvilinear array ultrasound probe with sterile cover and gel:

- Identify the vertebral spinous process
- Move laterally to the transverse process and costotransverse joint
- Then angle obliquely to identify the superior costotransverse ligament (hyperechoic)

In-plane technique, 18 G Touhy needle
Insert needle to make contact with the transverse process, then walk off it caudally (or cranially) to a level 10 mm deeper (may notice a slight loss of resistance)
After negative aspiration, slowly inject up to 20 ml of local anaesthetic (less if a multi-level approach is used)

Section 3

OSCE Stations 1–18 (Answers)

OSCE Station 15

Peripheral Nerves of the Upper Limb

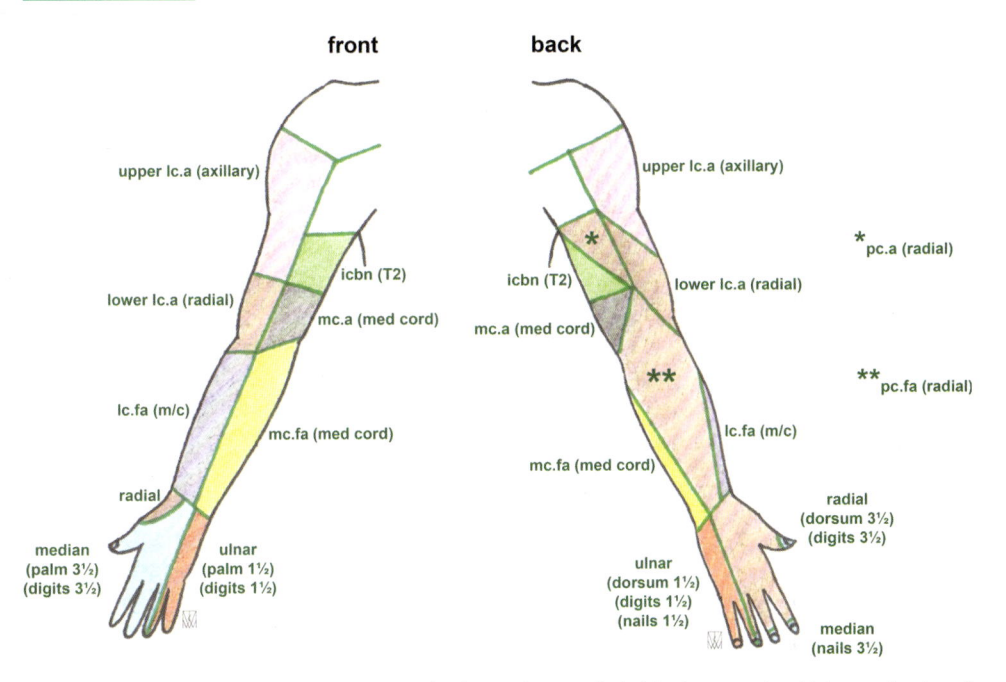

OSCE15 Upper limb nerves. Cutaneous nerve distribution in upper limb. **icbn** intercostobrachial nerve; **lc.a** lateral cutaneous nerve of arm; **lc.fa** lateral cutaneous nerve of forearm; **m/c** musculocutaneous; **mc.a** medial cutaneous nerve of arm; **mc.fa** medial cutaneous nerve of forearm; **pc.a** posterior cutaneous nerve of arm; **pc.fa** posterior cutaneous nerve of forearm.

a) Name the nerves that provide cutaneous innervation of the areas A–E in the diagram. Which one does not originate from the brachial plexus*? (6 marks)
   A) Lateral cutaneous nerve of the forearm (continuation of the musculocutaneous nerve)
   B) *Intercostobrachial nerve (the lateral cutaneous branch of T2 – not part of the brachial plexus)
   C) Median nerve
   D) Medial cutaneous nerve of the forearm
   E) Axillary nerve

b) Name two cutaneous branches of the radial nerve in the upper limb (2 marks)
   Posterior cutaneous nerve of the arm
   Inferior/lower lateral cutaneous nerve of the arm
   Posterior cutaneous nerve of the forearm
   Superficial branch of the radial nerve (terminal continuation of the radial nerve)

c) **Name three nerves with cutaneous innervation that may be blocked in the forearm? (3 marks)**

Median nerve (easiest to block in midforearm, lying between flexor digitorum superficialis and flexor digitorum profundus)

Radial nerve (superficial branch; most easily blocked just as it enters the forearm at the lateral aspect of the elbow/cubital fossa, lying between brachioradialis and brachial muscles)

Lateral cutaneous nerve of the forearm (continuation of the musculocutaneous nerve at the lateral border of the biceps tendon, runs with the cephalic vein)

Ulnar nerve (runs under flexor carpi ulnaris and approaches ulnar artery)

Medial cutaneous nerve of the forearm (less easy/reliable to identify, runs with the basilic vein)

d) **Name the muscle that overlies each of the following nerves in the midforearm (3 marks)**
Median nerve: flexor digitorum superficialis
Ulnar nerve: flexor carpi ulnaris
(Superficial branch of) radial nerve: brachioradialis

e) **Describe a technique for performing an ulnar nerve block in the midforearm**** (6 marks)**

Consent

Stop before you block: confirm side and site

SLIMRAG:

- Sterile procedure (wash hands, sterile gloves, sterile dressing pack)
- Light source/ultrasound
- IV access
- Monitoring (AAGBI minimum standard)
- Resuscitation drugs/equipment available
- Assistant (who is happy to assist with regional or general anaesthetic)
- General anaesthetic (ensure equipment/drugs available to convert if required)

Position: arm abducted, elbow flexed

Clean the skin with 0.5% chlorhexidine and allow to dry

High-frequency linear array transducer applied to the medial surface of the midforearm (with sterile cover and gel on probe)

Identify the nerve lying on the medial side of the ulnar artery at the wrist, then trace it proximally until it separates from the artery (to reduce the risk of vascular puncture)

At this point it lies directly beneath flexor carpi ulnaris

Local anaesthetic to skin, then in-plane technique: blunt 22 G 50-mm block needle from medial side of upper limb for in-plane approach (can also be done out of plane)

After negative aspiration, slowly inject 2–5 ml of local anaesthetic

**Avoid blocking the ulnar nerve behind the elbow (in the cubital tunnel) due to the risk of compressive neuropraxia

Section 3

OSCE Stations 1–18 (Answers)

OSCE Station 16

Rectus Abdominis, Sheath and Rectus Sheath Block

a.

b.

c.

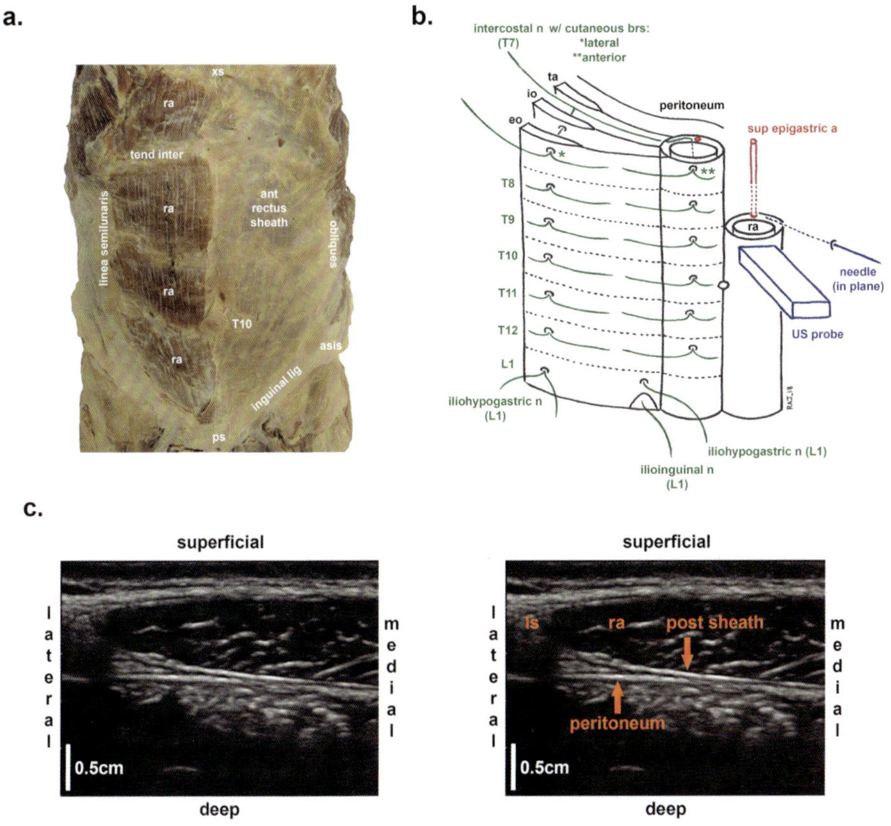

OSCE16 Anterior abdominal wall and rectus sheath block. a. Dissection of anterior abdominal wall. b. Schematic showing technique of rectus sheath block. c. US image during block. **asis** anterior superior iliac spine; **eo** external oblique; **io** internal oblique; **ls** linea semilunaris; **ps** pubic symphysis; **ra** rectus abdominis; **ta** transversus abdominis; **tend inter** tendinous intersection; **xs** xiphisternum.

a) Name the muscle in OSCE16, and describe its origin and insertion (3 marks)
   Rectus abdominis muscle
   Origin: pubic crest (lateral head) and pubic symphysis (medial head)
   Insertion: anterior surface of 5th, 6th and 7th costal cartilages

b) **At what level are the tendinous intersections (which give this muscle its classical appearance), and to which layer of the rectus sheath are they adherent? (2 marks)**
Upper: at the level of the xiphoid process
Middle: midway between xiphoid process and umbilicus
Lower: at the level of the umbilicus
Adherent to anterior layer of sheath (visible through skin of lean individuals – '6 pack')

c) **Describe the layers and contents of the rectus sheath (6 marks)**
Layers (in relation to rectus abdominis):
- Above costal margin:
  - Anterior: aponeurosis of external oblique only
  - Posterior: ribs/costal cartilages only (no sheath)
- Costal margin to arcuate line:
  - Anterior: aponeuroses of internal oblique (anterior lamella) and external oblique
  - Posterior: aponeuroses of internal oblique (posterior lamella) and transversus abdominis

Below arcuate line (around halfway between umbilicus and pubic symphysis):
- Anterior: aponeuroses of all three muscles
- Posterior: transversalis fascia (no sheath)

Contents:
- Rectus abdominis muscle (and pyramidalis muscle when present – around 80%)
- Superior and inferior (deep) epigastric arteries, with their accompanying veins
- T7–11 thoracoabdominal and T12 (subcostal) nerves, with their accompanying vessels (motor to rectus abdominis; sensory to parietal peritoneum, muscle and overlying skin)

d) **Describe the regions of the following dermatomes (3 marks)**
T10: umbilicus
L1: inguinal ligament
T7: xiphoid process

> **Block tips...**
> If inserting a rectus sheath catheter, an 18 G Tuohy needle provides excellent ultrasound visibility and allows passage of an appropriately sized catheter

e) **Describe how you would perform a rectus sheath block (6 marks)**
Consent
Stop before you block: confirm side and site (usually bilateral)
SLIMRAG:
- Sterile procedure (wash hands, sterile gloves, sterile dressing pack)
- Light source/ultrasound
- IV access
- Monitoring (AAGBI minimum standard)
- Resuscitation drugs/equipment available

OSCE Station 16: Rectus Abdominis, Sheath and Rectus Sheath Block

- Assistant (who is happy to assist with regional or general anaesthetic)
- General anaesthetic: ensure equipment/drugs available to convert if required

Position the patient supine, exposed from costal margin to inguinal ligament

Clean the field with 0.5% chlorhexidine (allow to dry)

High-frequency linear array ultrasound probe with sterile cover and gel

Place the probe in the midline (midway between the xiphisternum and umbilicus), aligned transversely, then scan laterally:

- Off the midline is the oval appearance of the rectus abdominis muscle
- Two echogenic layers on posterior surface: posterior rectus sheath and peritoneum (with intervening transversalis fascia appearing dark)

In-plane technique, 80-mm short-bevel regional block needle: inserted from lateral to medial, aiming for the needle tip to reach the potential space between the muscle and posterior wall of the rectus sheath

After negative aspiration, slowly inject 20–30 ml local anaesthetic on either side (depending on dose calculation), confirming negative aspiration after every 5-ml injection

Section 3: OSCE Stations 1–18 (Answers)

OSCE Station 17: Ribs and Ventilation

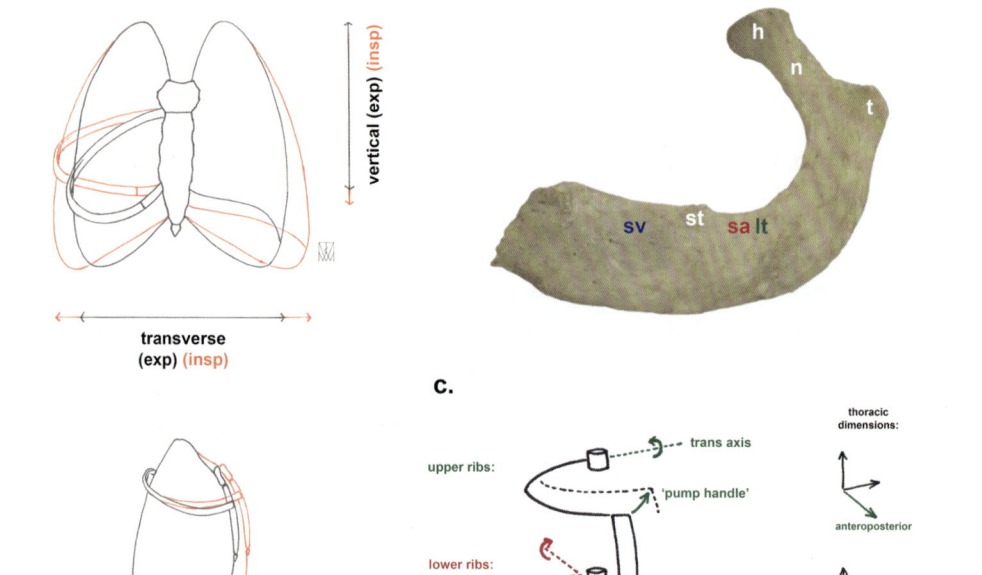

OSCE17 Ribs and ventilation. a. First rib. b. and c. Changes in the three thoracic dimensions during respiration. **h** head; **lt** groove for lower trunk of brachial plexus; **n** neck; **sa** groove for subclavian artery; **st** scalene tubercle; **sv** groove for subclavian vein; **t** tubercle/angle.

a) **What is meant by the term true, false and floating ribs? (6 marks)**

Relates to the anterior attachment of the rib/costal cartilage:

True ribs (1–7):
- Attach/articulate directly with the sternum/manubrium

False ribs (8–10):
- Articulate with the rib/costal cartilage immediately above (i.e. indirectly with the sternum)

Floating ribs (11–12):
- No anterior attachment (anterior end lies free in the body wall musculature)

b) **Identify the bone shown in OSCE17, and describe two ways of determining which side of the body it is from (3 marks)**

First rib

How to 'side' the bone:
- Scalene tubercle present on the superior surface of the shaft (for attachment of scalenus anterior)
- In the correct orientation, the rib should lie stable on a flat surface with each end touching the table, and the tubercle will be the most superior structure (and lies posteriorly)

c) **Describe five features of the first rib that are different from/not seen on a typical rib (5 marks)**

Singular articular surface on the head of the rib as atypical ribs (1, 11 and 12) articulate posteriorly with a single vertebra from its own level (i.e. rib 1 and T1) – typical ribs have two facets

Angle and tubercle of first rib are combined (typical ribs have separate angle and tubercle)

Flattened from top to bottom creating superior/inferior surfaces and medial/lateral borders (typical ribs are flattened from side to side, forming inner and outer surfaces with a smooth upper and sharp lower border)

Scalene tubercle present on the superior surface (not present on other ribs)

Grooves for the subclavian vein and artery/lower trunk of the brachial plexus (anterior and posterior to the scalene tubercle respectively)

Costal groove absent from under surface (present on typical ribs)

The anterior end forms a primary cartilaginous joint with the manubrium (this type of joint is called a synchondrosis (i.e. two bones with intervening hyaline cartilage), which only allows limited movement, thus providing a brace for the ribs below to 'pull up' against via the intercostal muscles*)

*Typical ribs articulate anteriorly with the sternum/rib above through synovial joints to allow movement during respiration

d) **Describe the movements that bring about spontaneous ('negative pressure') ventilation (6 marks)**

There are three 'diameters' to the thorax: anteroposterior, transverse and vertical

During inspiration these diameters increase, and lung volume expands (the lungs being held to the inside of the thoracic cage by the negative pressure in the pleural potential space)

This expansion is accompanied by a drop in pressure within the airspaces of the lungs, so air enters (the reverse holds true for expiration)

These changes are thus:
- Anteroposterior diameter: increased by the 'pump handle' movement, which raises the anterior end of the ribs (upper six ribs/most marked in ribs 2–6, axis of movement along neck of rib)

- Transverse diameter: increased by the 'bucket handle' movement, which raises the middle part of the ribs (lower six ribs/most marked in ribs 7–10, axis of movement ribs between the anterior/posterior ends of each rib)
- Vertical diameter: descent of the diaphragm as it contracts

Section 3: OSCE Stations 1–18 (Answers)

OSCE Station 18: Vertebrae and Spinal Ligaments

a.

cervical (w/ foramina transversaria) thoracic (w/ costal facets) lumbar (w/ neither ft or cf)

b.

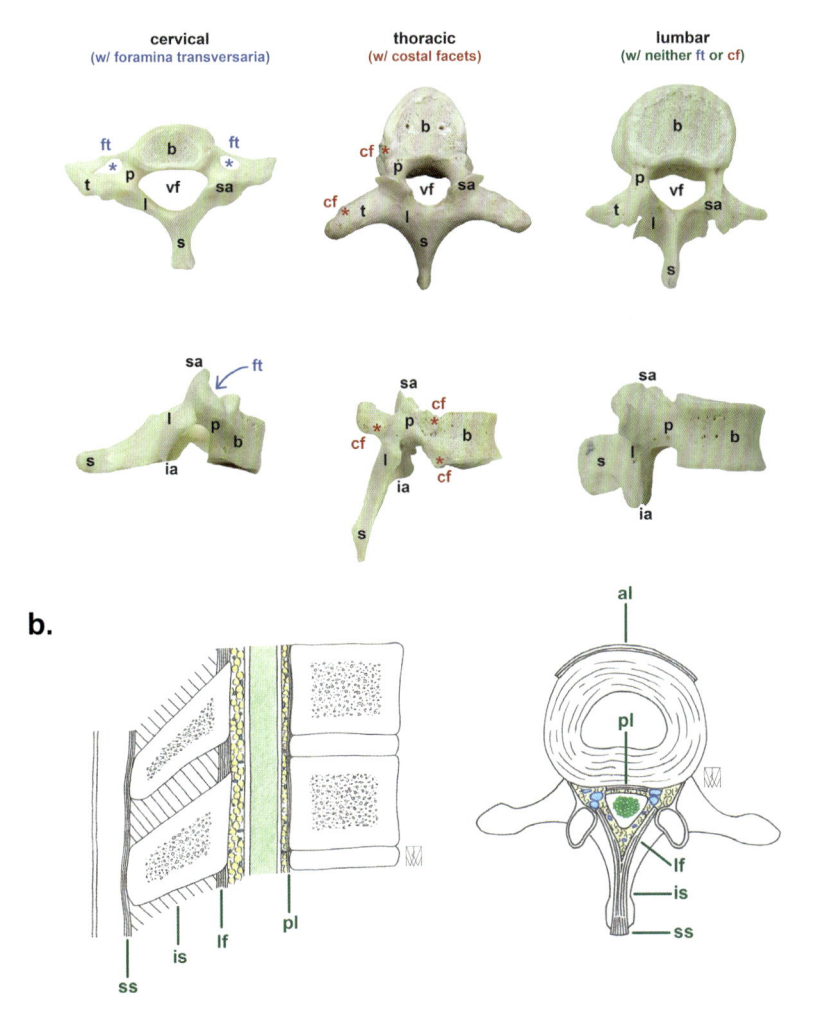

OSCE18 Vertebrae. a. Cervical, thoracic and lumbar vertebrae. b. Vertebral ligaments. **al** anterior longitudinal ligament; **b** body; **cf** costal facet; **ft** foramen transversarium; **ia** inferior articular process; **is** interspinous ligament; **l** lamina; **lf** ligamentum flavum; **p** pedicle; **pl** posterior longitudinal ligament; **s** spinous process; **sa** superior articular process; **ss** supraspinous ligament; **t** transverse process; **vf** vertebral foramen.

Section 3: OSCE Stations 1–18 (Answers)

a) **How many vertebrae are there in the cervical, thoracic and lumbar regions of the spine? (3 marks)**
 Cervical: 7
 Thoracic: 12
 Lumbar: 5

b) **From which regions of the spine do A, B and C originate? (3 marks)**
 A) Thoracic
 B) Lumbar
 C) Cervical

c) **What types of joint exist between vertebrae? (2 marks)**
 Secondary cartilaginous joint (between vertebral bodies – intervertebral discs)
 Synovial joint (between vertebral arches – the facet/zygapophyseal joint)

d) **Do the vertebrae articulate with any other structures? (2 marks)**
 Yes:
 - Ribs (costo-vertebral and costo-transverse joints; plane synovial joint)
 - Skull/occiput (atlanto-occipital joint; condyloid synovial joint)
 - Pelvis (sacroiliac joint; atypical synovial joint)

e) **Name structures 1–4 (4 marks)**
 1) Interspinous ligament
 2) Ligamentum flavum
 3) Supraspinous ligament
 4) Posterior longitudinal ligament

f) **Which areas of the spinal column are most commonly fractured and why? (3 marks)**
 Cervical (particularly C7; C5/6 commonest level of spinal cord damage)
 Lumbar (T12, L1/2)
 Both are regions where areas of mobile spine (cervical and lumbar) adjoin an immobile area (thoracic)

g) **What techniques could you employ to intubate a patient with an unstable cervical spine fracture? (3 marks)**
 Awake fibre-optic intubation
 Awake videolaryngoscopy
 Asleep fibre-optic intubation (+/− LMA/ILMA)
 Asleep laryngoscopy with cervical spine immobilisation
 Awake tracheostomy

Section 4

SOEs 1–3 (Answers)

SOE 1a

Cervical Plexus and Carotid Endarterectomy

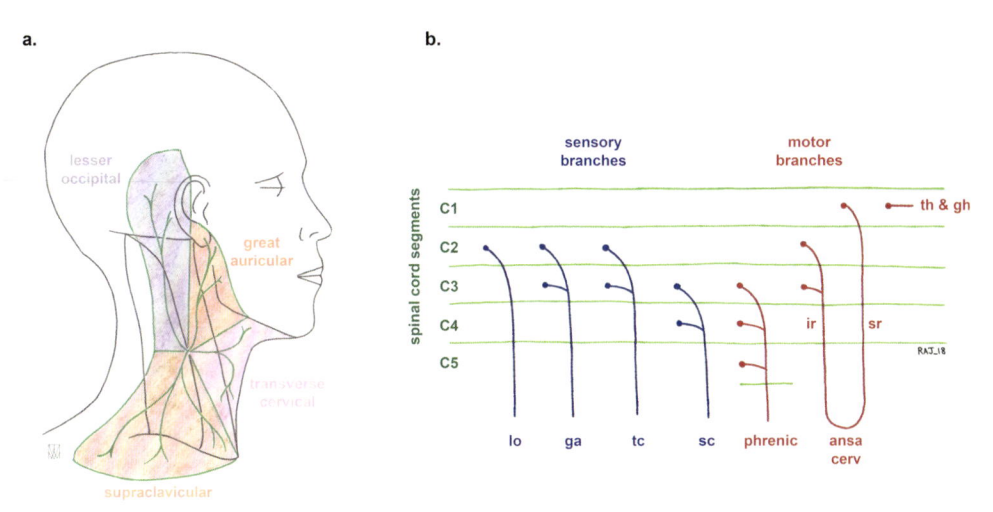

a.

b.

SOE1a Cervical plexus a. Distribution of cutaneous branches of cervical plexus. b. Schematic of cervical plexus. The ansa cervicalis supplies the strap muscles. **ansa cerv** ansa cervicalis; **ga** great auricular; **ir** inferior root; **lo** lesser occipital; **sc** supraclavicular; **sr** superior root; **tc** transverse cervical; **th & gh** thyrohyoid & geniohyoid.

a) **How can anaesthesia for carotid end arterectomy be provided?**
   Local anaesthetic infiltration
   Cervical epidural
   Cervical plexus block:
   - Deep
   - Deep and superficial
   - Superficial and local anaesthetic infiltration

   General anaesthetic

b) **What nerve roots contribute to the cervical plexus, and where does this plexus lie?**
   Formed by branches of anterior rami of C1–4 (after they have received grey rami communicantes from the superior cervical ganglion)
   Lies on scalenus medius (deep to prevertebral fascia)

c) **Name the cutaneous branches of the cervical plexus (aka superficial cervical plexus) and describe their sensory distribution**

Nerves emerge at the posterior border of sternocleidomastoid and pierce deep investing fascia of the neck midway between mastoid process and sternal notch (just below CN 11)

Lesser occipital nerve (C2):
- Runs obliquely up along the posterior border of sternocleidomastoid
- Supplies scalp behind the auricle

Great auricular nerve (C2/3)*:
- Runs straight up over the belly of sternocleidomastoid
- Supplies skin over the cranial surface of the auricle, the external auditory meatus and lateral surface of auricle below this, also supplies angle of mandible and parotid gland/fascia

Transverse cervical nerve (C2/3):
- Travels anteriorly and divides into superior and inferior branches
- Supplies skin from chin/margin of mandible to sternal angle

Supraclavicular nerve (C3/4):
- Runs a short course before dividing into three main groups of branches
  - Medial group: supplies skin from the midline to the anterior shoulder, as far inferiorly as the sternal angle/second rib
  - Intermediate group: supplies skin over the proximal half way of deltoid muscle
  - Lateral group: supplies skin across the acromion posteriorly down to the spine of the scapula

*There is no *greater* auricular nerve! However, this is frequently referred to in texts

d) **Compare and contrast general and regional techniques of anaesthesia for carotid endarterectomy**

General:
- Advantages:
  - Patient may prefer GA
  - Secure airway, control ventilation
  - Reduced cerebral metabolic rate of oxygen consumption
  - Removes time constraints of blocks and minimises issues with patient compliance in prolonged cases
  - No need for intraoperative local anaesthesia supplementation
- Disadvantages:
  - Cardiovascular instability of GA
  - Removes option of gold standard cerebral blood flow monitoring (patient interaction)
  - Higher rate of shunt use
  - GA may influence neurological/cognitive status/ability to assess postoperatively

Regional:
- Advantages:
  - Maintains cardiovascular stability (both intra- and postoperatively)
  - Preservation of cerebral autoregulation
  - Allows continuous monitoring of cerebral blood flow/neurological function
  - Lower rate of shunt use
  - Allows earlier assessment of postoperative neurological function
- Disadvantages:
  - Conversion to GA intraoperatively may be more difficult than preoperatively
  - Requires patient compliance
  - Surgical team may not be happy with awake patient
  - Higher BP intraoperatively
  - Patient preference/claustrophobia with drapes
  - Patient movement: coughing, shivering if cold, restlessness/need to micturate
  - Potential complications from regional anaesthesia technique

There does not seem to be strong evidence for the superiority of one technique over another – hence why the debate exists!

Section 4 — SOE 1b

Anterolateral Abdominal Wall and TAP Block

SOEs 1–3 (Answers)

a.

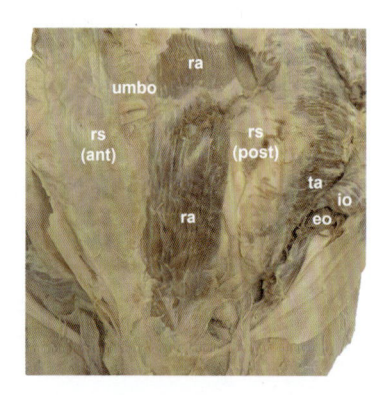

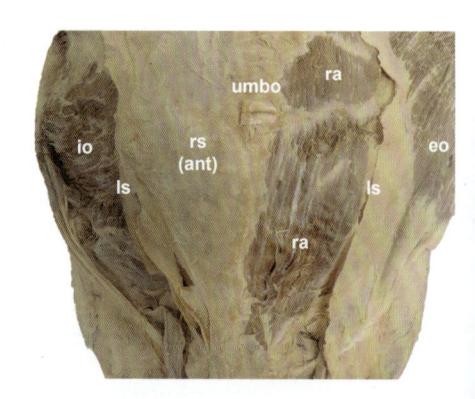

b.

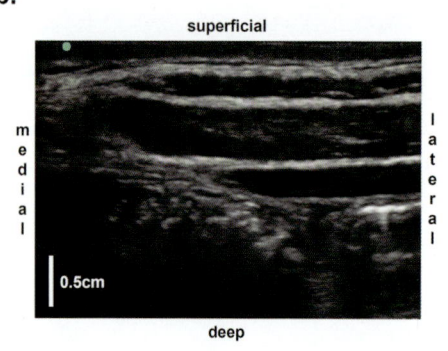

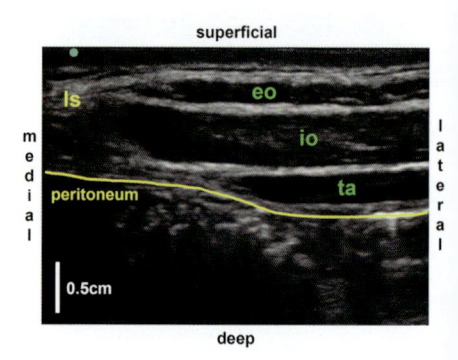

SOE1b Anterolateral abdominal wall and TAP block a. Dissection of anterolateral abdominal wall muscles to show the three layers of the body wall. b. US image of the three layers – external oblique, internal oblique and transversus abdominis. **eo** external oblique; **io** internal oblique; **ls** linea semilunaris; **ra** rectus abdominis; **rs (ant)** rectus sheath (anterior); **rs (post)** rectus sheath (posterior); **ta** transversus abdominis; **umbo** umbilicus.

a) On the ultrasound image SOE1b, identify the muscles of the anterolateral abdominal wall (excluding rectus abdominis) and describe the orientation of their fibres
   External oblique muscle (EO; fibres pass downwards and forwards, 'hands in pockets' orientation)
   Internal oblique muscle (IO; fibres pass upwards and forwards, perpendicular to EO)
   Transversus abdominis muscle (TA; fibres pass transversely forwards to meet in the midline)

b) **Describe their origin and insertion**
   External oblique:
   - Origin: lower eight ribs
   - Insertion: linea alba (via rectus sheath), pubic tubercle and anterior half of iliac crest (lower margin of EO aponeurosis between pubic tubercle and ASIS forms the inguinal ligament)

   Internal oblique:
   - Origin: thoracolumbar fascia (TFL), anterior two-thirds of iliac crest and lateral two-thirds of inguinal ligament
   - Insertion: costal margin, linea alba (via rectus sheath), pubic crest (pectineal line via the conjoint tendon)

   Transversus abdominis (TA):
   - Origin: costal margin, TFL, anterior two-thirds of iliac crest and lateral one-third of inguinal ligament
   - Insertion: linea alba (via rectus sheath), pubic crest (pectineal line via the conjoint tendon)

c) **In which plane does the main neurovascular bundle lie? What nerves are found here?**
   Plane: deep to IO and superficial to TA (i.e. between the middle and inner layers of the anterolateral abdominal wall)
   Nerves:
   - Thoracoabdominal nerves: T7–11
   - Subcostal nerve: T12
   - Iliohypogastric nerve and its collateral branch (ilioinguinal nerve): L1

d) **For which types of surgery may a transversus abdominis plane (TAP) block be beneficial?**
   Lower abdominal surgery (around umbilicus (T9/10) and below; open inguinal/umbilical hernia repair, open appendicectomy, lower midline laparotomy)
   Gynaecological/obstetric surgery (abdominal hysterectomy, caesarian section)
   Urology (e.g. prostatectomy, nephrectomy, renal transplant)

e) **Describe how you would perform a TAP block**
   Consent
   Stop before you block (confirm side and site if unilateral)
   SLIMRAG:
   - Sterile procedure (wash hands, sterile gloves, sterile dressing pack)
   - Light source/ultrasound
   - IV access
   - Monitoring (AAGBI minimum standard)
   - Resuscitation drugs/equipment available
   - Assistant (who is happy to assist with regional or general anaesthetic)
   - General anaesthetic: ensure equipment/drugs available to convert if required

   Position the patient supine, exposed from costal margin to below the iliac crest
   Clean the field with 0.5% chlorhexidine and allow to dry
   High-frequency linear array ultrasound probe with sterile cover and gel

Place the probe in the midline, aligned transversely, then scan laterally/posteriorly to the midaxillary line (between the costal margin and iliac crest):
- Off the midline is the oval appearance of the rectus abdominis muscle
- At its lateral border (linear semilunaris) are the three muscles of the lateral wall (EO, IO and TA)
- Moving further laterally, these muscles will be visible as three parallel layers

In-plane technique with 80- to 100-mm short-bevel regional block needle (inserted anteriorly, directed posterolaterally)

After negative aspiration, inject 20 ml local anaesthetic on one/both sides, confirming negative aspiration after every 5-ml injection

Confirm local anaesthetic spread within the plane between IO and TA during injection

Section 4

SOE 1c

SOEs 1–3 (Answers)

Brachial Plexus and Interscalene Block

a.

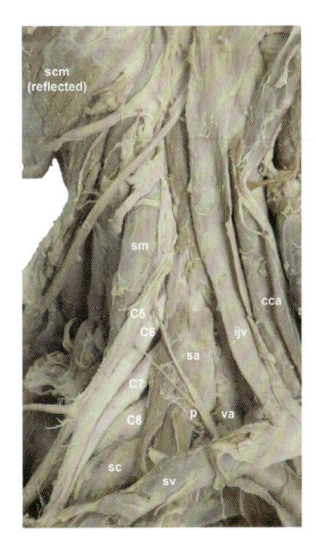

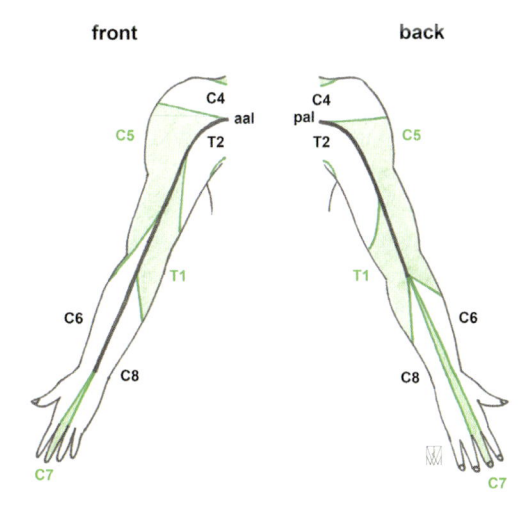

b.

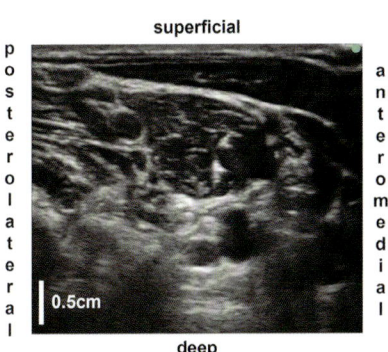

c.

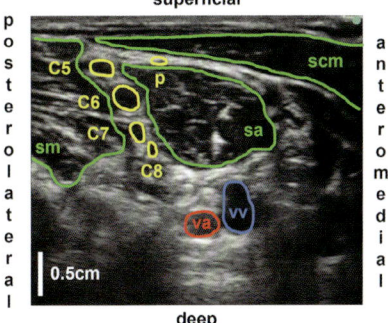

SOE1c Brachial plexus and interscalene block a. Dissection of neck to show roots of brachial plexus emerging between scalenus anterior and scalenus medius. b. US image of same region. c. Segmental/dermatomal supply of upper limb. **aal** anterior axial line; **cca** common carotid artery; **ijv** internal jugular vein; **p** phrenic nerve; **pal** posterior axial line; **sa** scalenus anterior; **sc** subclavian artery; **scm** sternocleidomastoid; **sm** scalenus medius; **sv** subclavian vein; **va** vertebral artery; **vv** vertebral vein.

Section 4: SOEs 1–3 (Answers)

a) **On the right-hand image of SOE1c, label the dermatomes of the upper limb**
   (C4 – acromioclavicular joint/shoulder tip)
   C5 – lateral arm
   C6 – lateral forearm, thumb and index finger
   C7 – middle finger
   C8 – ring/little finger and medial forearm
   T1 – medial arm
   (T2 – axilla)

b) **What peripheral nerves supply the shoulder joint and skin of the shoulder region? Describe the region they supply**
   (Lateral) supraclavicular nerve (C3/4): skin over shoulder as far as clavicle (anteriorly), acromion (laterally) and spine of scapula (posteriorly)
   Suprascapular nerve (C5/6): acromioclavicular joint/capsule and shoulder joint
   Axillary nerve (C5/6): shoulder joint and 'regimental badge' area
   Musculocutaneous nerve (C5/6/7): shoulder joint (and lateral forearm)
   Lateral pectoral nerve (C5/6/7): variable innervation around anterior shoulder joint soft tissue

c) **What regional anaesthesia technique may be performed to block these nerves, and which areas of the upper limb may not be blocked with this technique?**
   Interscalene brachial plexus block* is the most common technique (blocks proximal nerve roots of brachial plexus and distal cervical plexus – supraclavicular nerves)
   Areas missed:
   - Posterior shoulder (supraclavicular nerve: this area often must be augmented by local anaesthetic infiltration at the posterior port site for awake arthroscopic shoulder surgery)
   - Ring/little finger, medial forearm/arm and axilla (C8–T2: inferior roots of brachial plexus are not as well visualised in the interscalene grove and therefore may be missed, often blockade here is not required)

   *A shoulder block has also been described:
   - Separate axillary and suprascapular nerve blocks
   - Avoids phrenic nerve block and therefore may be useful in patient with significant respiratory limitation

d) **Name structures A–F on the ultrasound image in SOE1c of the interscalene groove**
   A) Nerve roots (C5–7)
   B) Scalenus anterior muscle
   C) Vertebral artery
   D) Sternocleidomastoid muscle
   E) Scalenus medius muscle
   F) Phrenic nerve

e) **List the possible neurological complications of an interscalene block**
   Cervical cord injury (by needle trauma/injection)
   Epidural/subarachnoid injection of local anaesthesia
   Phrenic nerve blockade (approaching 100% in high-volume block, symptomatic in around 30%)

Cervical sympathetic chain block (Horner's syndrome)
Vagal nerve block/injury or recurrent laryngeal nerve block/injury
Injury to nerve roots of brachial plexus
There is some concern that, using an in-plane technique, the dorsal scapular nerve and long thoracic nerves can be damaged by direct needle trauma as they lie on scalenus medius
Vascular trauma (vertebral artery): bleeding and intravascular injection/toxicity/seizure

Section 4 — SOE 1d

SOEs 1–3 (Answers)

Spinal Cord Blood Supply and Tracts

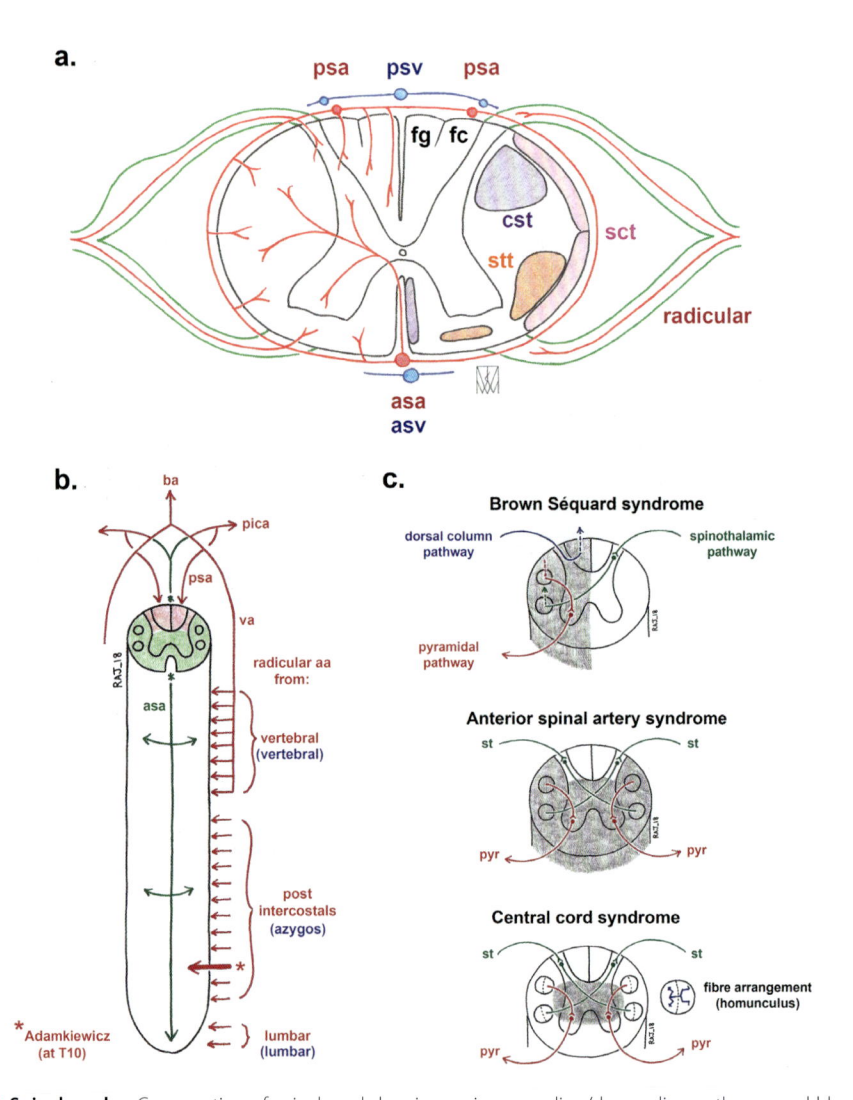

SOE1d Spinal cord. a. Cross-section of spinal cord showing major ascending/descending pathways and blood supply. Note that the radicular arteries anastomose variably with the anterior and posterior spinal arteries. b. Schematic of spinal cord to show origin and drainage of radicular vessels. c. Spinal cord syndromes. **asa** anterior spinal artery; **asv** anterior spinal vein; **ba** basilar artery; **cst** corticospinal tract; **fc** fasciculus cuneatus; **fg** fasciculus gracilis; **pica** posterior inferior cerebellar artery; **psa** posterior spinal artery; **psv** posterior spinal vein; **pyr** pyramidal pathway; **sct** spinocerebellar tract; **st** spinothalamic pathway; **stt** spinothalamic tract; **va** vertebral artery.

SOE 1d: Spinal Cord Blood Supply and Tracts

a) **Describe the blood supply to the spinal cord**
   Single anterior spinal artery:
   - Formed from the union of a branch of each vertebral artery at the foramen magnum
   - Descends whole length of spinal cord in anterior median fissure
   - Gives series of circumferential and central branches
   - Supplies anterior two-thirds of spinal cord: all of cord anterior to posterior grey columns

   Two posterior spinal arteries:
   - From posterior inferior cerebellar artery (75%) or vertebral artery (25%) at foramen magnum
   - Usually double on each side; trunks run through and behind posterior nerve rootlets for whole length of the cord

   Radicular arteries:
   - Important contribution as the longitudinal arteries (above) are variable in size
   - Anastomosing with and reinforce anterior and posterior spinal arteries
   - Arise from vertebral, posterior intercostal, lumbar and lateral sacral arteries
   - Enter through intervertebral foramina as spinal arteries
   - Penetrate meninges and run along nerve roots
   - Variable in number; not present at all levels
   - Largest: arteria radicularis magna (artery of Adamkiewicz), usually from lower intercostal or upper lumbar artery (T8–L3), on the left in 80% (in 15% arises at T5)

   Spinal veins:
   - One anterior spinal vein, one posterior spinal vein (on posterior median sulcus) and two posterolateral spinal veins (lateral to posterior spinal arteries)
   - Drain via internal vertebral venous plexus to external vertebral venous plexus, and then to vertebral, azygos, lumbar and lateral sacral veins

b) **Where are the 'watershed areas' in relation to blood supply of the spinal cord?**
   Found at junctions of cervical, thoracic and lumbar regions of cord, where the blood supply is tenuous and the cord is vulnerable to ischaemia (particularly at T4/5)

c) **On the illustration SOE1d, label the main ascending and descending tracts in the spinal cord, and describe the signals they transmit**
   Ascending:
   - Anterior (direct) and *lateral (crossed)* spinothalamic tracts (pain, temperature, touch)
   - Dorsal column-medial lemniscal: fasciculus cuneatus (C1–T6) and gracilis (T7 and below) (vibration, proprioception, touch)
   - Anterior and posterior spinocerebellar (unconscious proprioception: muscle length/tension)

   Descending:
   - Anterior (direct) and *lateral (crossed)* corticospinal tracts (voluntary movement)

d) **Which surgical procedures are associated with spinal cord ischaemia?**
   Aortic aneurysm repair (particularly thoracoabdominal)
   Aortic dissection
   Scoliosis surgery
   Laminectomy/spinal decompression
   Procedures causing periods of significant hypotension

e) **How can you prevent intraoperative spinal cord ischaemia?**
   Maintain adequate MAP:
   - Judicious monitoring (e.g. arterial line)
   - Appropriate use of IV fluids and vasoconstrictors/inotropes

   CSF drain (to reduce CSF pressure and increase spinal cord perfusion)
   Minimise duration of aortic cross-clamp
   Consider cardiopulmonary bypass or deep hypothermic circulatory arrest
   Monitoring of somatosensory evoked potentials
   Intrathecal vasodilators (e.g. papaverine), systemic Ca^{2+} channel blockers

Section 4 — SOEs 1–3 (Answers)

SOE 2a — Trigeminal Nerve (CN 5) and Trigeminal Neuralgia

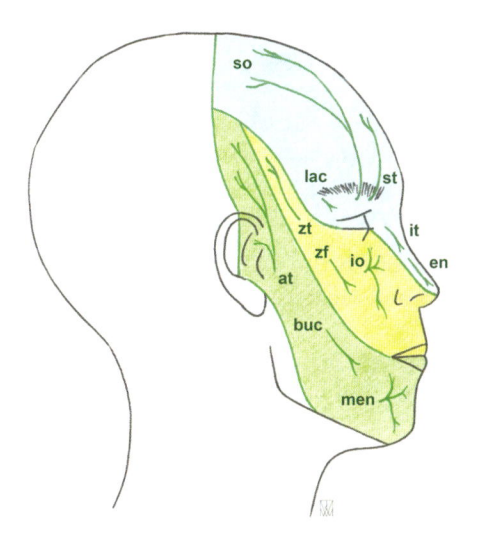

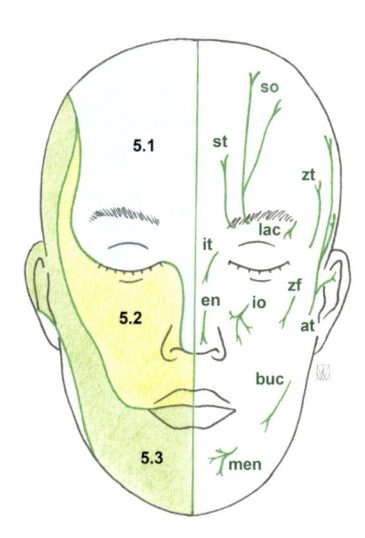

SOE2a Trigeminal nerve. Cutaneous supply of face and scalp. The three divisions of the trigeminal nerve are shown, along with the individual named branches. **at** auriculotemporal; **buc** buccal; **en** external nasal; **io** infraorbital; **it** infratrochlear; **lac** lacrimal; **men** mental; **so** supraorbital; **st** supratrochlear; **zf** zygomaticofacial; **zt** zygomaticotemporal.

a) **Describe the anatomy of the trigeminal nerve (CN 5)**

Single motor nucleus:
- Trigeminal motor nucleus (pons; motor to muscles of mastication and four others*)

Three sensory nuclei:
- Trigeminal mesencephalic nucleus (midbrain; proprioception)
- Trigeminal pontine (principal) nucleus (pons; touch)
- Trigeminal spinal nucleus (medulla; pain/temperature)

Arises from the pons as a large sensory root and a smaller motor root

The majority of sensory fibres have their cell body located in the trigeminal ganglion** (aka semilunar/Gasserian ganglion), lying within an evagination of arachnoid dura (cavum trigeminale/Meckel's cave) near the apex of the petrous temporal bone in the middle cranial fossa

Three sensory branches emerge:
- V1 (ophthalmic): passes forwards in lateral wall of cavernous sinus, divides into lacrimal, frontal (further divides: supraorbital and supratrochlear) and nasociliary branches, which exit middle cranial fossa through superior orbital fissure
- V2 (maxillary): passes forwards in lateral wall of cavernous sinus, leaves middle cranial fossa through foramen rotundum
- V3 (mandibular): passes inferiorly through foramen ovale, then joined by motor root to form a trunk that splits into two divisions (anterior is mainly motor and posterior is mainly sensory)

*Muscles supplied by CN 5:
- Muscles of mastication: masseter, temporalis, medial pterygoid, lateral pterygoid
- Four others: tensor tympani, tensor palati, anterior belly of digastric, mylohyoid

**Equivalent to the dorsal root ganglion of a spinal nerve

b) **Draw a diagram to describe the sensory supply of CN 5**
Sensation to face and scalp, from chin to vertex and ear to ear (but not angle of jaw)
Anterior meninges (dura and arachnoid)
Eye, nasal and oral cavities (including inside of cheek, mandible, teeth and gums)
General sensation to anterior two-thirds of tongue (but not taste***)

***Supplied by chorda tympani of CN 7

c) **What is trigeminal neuralgia (TN)?**
Episodic, severe, lancinating pain in CN 5 territory (V1/V2 more common, V3 rare)
Always unilateral, typically abrupt onset/offset
May develop allodynia or hyperalgesia (but no other neurological deficit)
Usually asymptomatic between paroxysms
May be no clear cause, but have various triggers (e.g. touch, shaving)
International Headache Society diagnostic criteria (ICHS Classification ICHD-3):
- Recurrent paroxysms of unilateral facial pain in the distribution of one or more division of CN 5, with no radiation beyond, and fulfilling the following criteria:
    - A: lasting up to two minutes + severe + electric shock-like/stabbing/sharp (duration can change over time)
    - B: triggered by innocuous stimuli within the CN 5 distribution (attacks can be/may appear to be spontaneous, but must be a history of pain provoked by stimuli)
    - C: not better accounted for by another ICHD-3 diagnosis

d) **What are the risk factors and how is the diagnosis made?**
Risk factors:
- Female (F:M 2:1)
- Age (rare before 50 years, peak onset 60–70 years)
- Occurs in 3–4% of patients with multiple sclerosis (MS) (often in younger patients)

- There is an association with hypertension
- Possibly a familial link (suggested to be a result of inherited blood vessel malformation)

Diagnosis:
- Clinical, from the history
- MRI can help exclude brainstem lesion and vascular malformation

e) **What causes TN?**
Unclear
Primary/secondary demyelination of CN 5 leads to uncontrolled firing of small fibres (e.g. secondary demyelination due to compression by one of the cerebellar arteries)
Occurs partly because of lack of inhibitory input from large myelinated fibres (e.g. in MS, due to blood vessel compressing nerve)
Central mechanism also suggested

f) **Describe the management of TN**
Conservative
- Psychological support may be important for resistance/poorly responsive cases

Medical
- Cabamazepine (effective in >90%, if no response reconsider diagnosis)
- Phenytoin second line
- Other agents: gabapentin, amitriptyline, baclofen, clonazepam, lamotrigine

Surgical/interventional
- Alcohol injection at various points along the nerve (now rarely performed)
- Glycerol injection of the trigeminal ganglion (both aim to selectively destroy pain fibres, glycerol technique has higher success rate)
- Balloon decompression (destroying sensory fibres)
- Gamma knife techniques (stereotactic-guided radio-ablation: needle passed through foramen ovale into trigeminal ganglion, benefit may take months to develop)
- Open microvascular decompression of CN 5 (effective in >80%, previously only done if imaging demonstrated a vessel compressing the nerve, but may be effective even if preoperative imaging does not show this)

Section 4 — SOEs 1–3 (Answers)

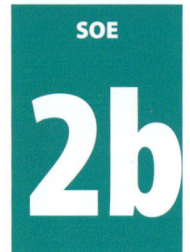

SOE 2b: Pleura and Interpleural Block

a.

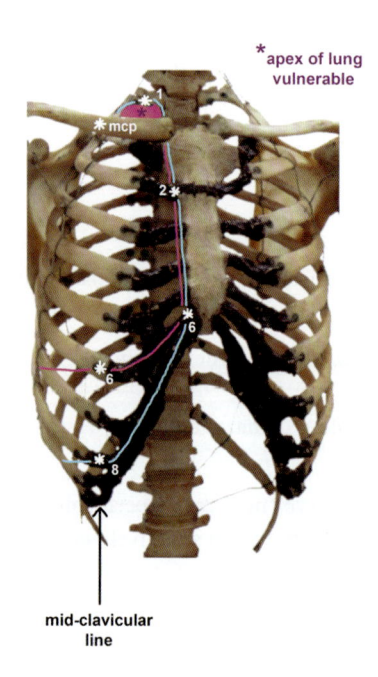

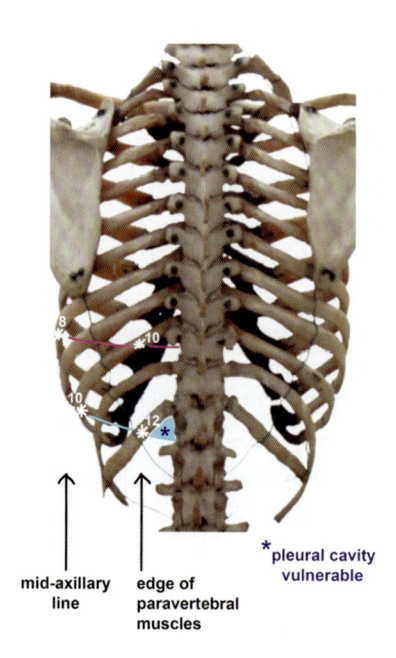

*apex of lung vulnerable

*mcp

mid-clavicular line

mid-axillary line

edge of paravertebral muscles

*pleural cavity vulnerable

b.

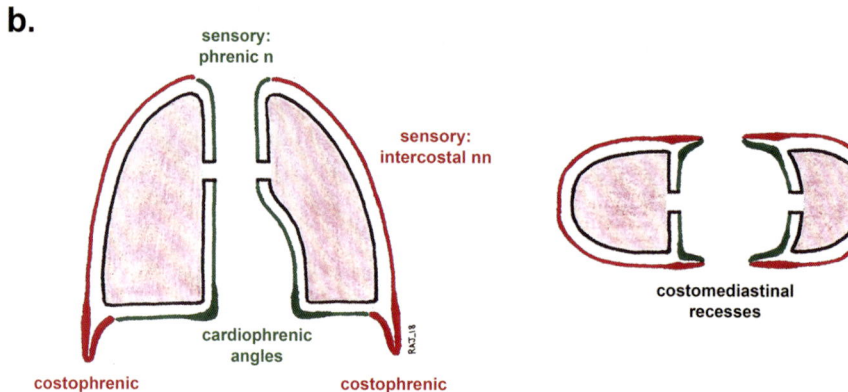

sensory: phrenic n

sensory: intercostal nn

cardiophrenic angles

costophrenic recess

costophrenic recess

costomediastinal recesses

SOE2b Pleura. a. Surface markings of pleura (blue) and lungs (red) superimposed on thoracic cage. Note the vulnerable parts of the lung and pleural cavity. b. Pleural recesses. Sensory supply of parietal pleura. **mcp** midclavicular point.

SOE 2b: Pleura and Interpleural Block

a) **What are the pleural membranes and where are they found?**
   Pair of serous membranes (thin membrane of fibrous tissue with single layer of squamous cells; mesothelium)
   Parietal pleura:
   - Lines inner surface of the thorax, mediastinum and upper surface of the diaphragm
   - Bound to inner surface of thoracic cage by endothoracic fascia
   - Bound superiorly at thoracic inlet to suprapleural membrane (Sibson's fascia)

   Visceral pleura covers the surface of each lung (including fissures)
   Parietal and visceral pleura are in contact and lubricated by a thin film of tissue fluid

b) **Describe the surface markings of the pleura with reference to the photograph of the thoracic skeleton***
   2.5 cm above the junction of the middle and medial thirds of the clavicle (but not above the neck of the first rib)
   In the midline at the **2nd** rib (sternal angle)
   At **4th** costal cartilage:
   - Right side continues vertically down
   - Left side sweeps out and descends behind the costal cartilages

   Both pleura pass behind the **6th** costal cartilage
   Midclavicular line: **8th** costal cartilage
   Midaxillary line: **10th** rib
   Midscapular line (lateral border of erector spinae): **12th** rib
   Passes horizontally to the lower border of **T12**
   (Note that a triangle of pleura lies below the medial part of the 12th rib)

*Easy: 2–4–6–8–10–12!
(See bold numbers in text)

c) **What are the costodiaphragmatic and costomediastinal recesses and where are they found**?**
   The lungs only occupy the full space indicated by the surface markings of the pleura at the peak of inspiration
   At other times, below the inferior border of the lung the costal and diaphragmatic parietal pleura are in contact (separated by a thin layer of tissue fluid)
   The potential space found here is the costodiaphragmatic recess
   The same is true of the potential space between the costal and mediastinal parietal pleura anteriorly

**The lungs don't always occupy the whole pleural space, creating recesses:
- The anterior borders of the lungs are similar (apart from a slightly larger 'cardiac notch' for the left lung)
- 6th costal cartilage in midclavicular line
- 8th rib in midaxillary line
- 10th rib in midscapular line
- Pass medially to T10

d) **Describe the innervation of the pleura**
   Parietal:
   - Intercostal nerves supply the costal and peripheral diaphragmatic parts
   - Phrenic nerve supplies mediastinal parts and central portion of the diaphragmatic parts

   Visceral:
   - Sympathetic nociception and vasomotor

e) **What are the indications for an interpleural block?**
   Surgery (thoracotomy, chest wall surgery, upper abdominal laparotomy)
   Trauma (analgesia for rib fractures, chest drain insertion)
   Chronic pain (post herpetic neuralgia, cancer pain, pancreatitis)

f) **Outline how to perform an interpleural block**
   Consent
   Stop before you block: confirm side and site
   SLIMRAG:
   - Sterile procedure (wash hands, sterile gloves, sterile dressing pack)
   - Light source/ultrasound
   - IV access
   - Monitoring (AAGBI minimum standard)
   - Resuscitation drugs/equipment available
   - Assistant (who is happy to assist with regional or general anaesthetic)
   - General anaesthetic (ensure equipment/drugs available to convert if required)

   Equipment: 16 G Tuohy needle connected to a three-way tap and a bag of normal saline
   Position the patient (supine or lateral, flat or semirecumbent)
   Clean skin with 0.5% chlorhexidine (allow to dry)
   Local anaesthetic to skin
   Needle insertion point (various described):
   - Anterior/mid/posterior axillary line or 10 cm from dorsal midline, in the 4th to 8th intercostal space
   - Midclavicular line, 2nd intercostal space
   - Avoid the neurovascular bundle below the rib (N.B. there is also a lesser neurovascular bundle above each rib)

   Insert Tuohy needle through skin and connective tissue until contact is made with the rib
   Open three-way tap to bag of fluid
   Advance the needle during expiration (spontaneously breathing patient) or at the end of expiration with the ventilator disconnected (mechanically ventilated patient)
   Walk the needle off the superior border of the rib
   Advance the needle until fluid runs freely from the bag of saline (thus identifying the negative pressure of the interpleural space)
   Open three-way tap to inject local anaesthetic (e.g. 30 ml 0.25% L-bupivacaine) into the interpleural space
   (Insert catheter if required)
   Withdraw the needle

Section 4

SOEs 1–3 (Answers)

SOE 2c: Cubital Fossa and Inadvertent Intra-Arterial Injection

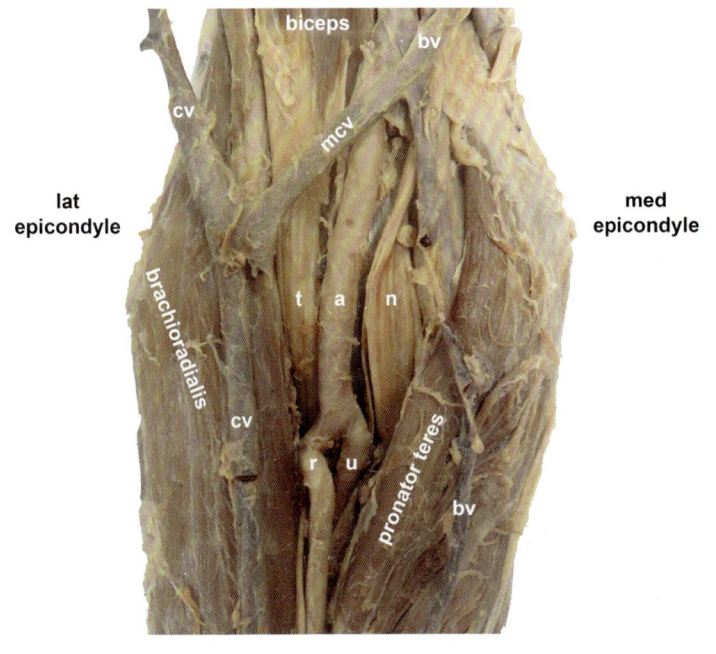

SOE2c Cubital fossa. Dissection of right cubital fossa – note order of structures ('t a n'). **a** brachial artery; **bv** basilic vein; **cv** cephalic vein; **mcv** median cubital vein; **n** median nerve; **r** radial artery; **t** tendon of biceps brachii; **u** ulnar artery.

a) Describe the boundaries of the cubital fossa with reference to the cadaveric image SOE2c
   Proximal: line joining the medial and lateral epicondyles of the humerus
   Inferolateral: medial border of brachioradialis
   Inferomedial: lateral border of pronator teres
   Roof: deep fascia of forearm (reinforced by the bicipital aponeurosis)
   Floor: brachialis, capsule of elbow joint, supinator muscle

Section 4: SOEs 1–3 (Answers)

b) **What are the contents of the cubital fossa?***
Biceps tendon
Brachial artery (dividing into radial and ulnar arteries)
Median nerve

*TAN:
- Tendon
- Artery
- Nerve

The radial nerve is included in some descriptions, lying between brachioradialis and brachialis

c) **Name the superficial veins associated with the cubital fossa, the areas they drain and where they drain to**
Cephalic (drains lateral side of forearm, runs up lateral edge of biceps to deltopectoral groove and pierces clavipectoral fascia to drain into the axillary vein)
Basilic (drains medial side of forearm, runs up medial side of arm and pierces deep fascia half way up the arm, to join the venae commitantes of the brachial artery and form the axillary vein at the inferior border of teres major)
Median cubital (connects cephalic and basilic veins, lies over the bicipital aponeurosis)
Variations in the pattern of these veins are common

d) **What are the features of inadvertent intra-arterial injection here?**
May be asymptomatic
The drug may fail to elicit the expected effect
Pain and paraesthesia (if patient awake) in the hand
Ischaemic changes (vasospasm): cool, pale, mottled, cyanosed
May be unable to feel distal pulses (may ultimately develop oedema and tissue necrosis)

e) **Why is intra-arterial injection of thiopentone problematic?**
Thiopentone is a thiobarbiturate that demonstrates structural isomerism (molecules have same molecular formula but differ in the order in which the elements are arranged)
In solution it has a pH of 10.4: at this pH it exists as the enol form, which is water soluble
The pKa of thiopentone is 7.6
Therefore, at physiological pH 7.34–7.45 it transforms into the keto form, which is fat soluble and acid crystals precipitate out of solution
When injected into a vein, this is not significant because the crystals are subject to serial dilution as the blood mixes with that from other veins
When injected into an artery, the crystals can occlude the vessel and cause intense vasospasm

f) **How would you manage a patient who has just received inadvertent intra-arterial injection of thiopentone?**
No universally agreed protocol: aim to maintain distal perfusion
Stop injection
Maintain the arterial cannula in place
500 ml warmed fluids through the cannula can dilute the crystals

SOE 2c: Cubital Fossa and Inadvertent Intra-Arterial Injection

Intra-arterial injection of 1% lignocaine may provide analgesia
500–1000 units heparin through the cannula to reduce the risk of thrombosis
Treat arterial spasm with papaverine (smooth muscle relaxant), prostacyclin, tolazoline (noradrenaline antagonist) or phenoxybenzamine (alpha 1 antagonist)
Can consider stellate ganglion/brachial plexus block to achieve vasodilation/analgesia
May need to maintain heparinisation for up to 14 days

Section 4 SOEs 1–3 (Answers)

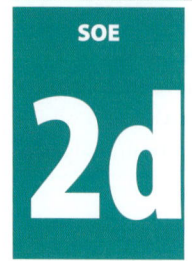

SOE 2d — Sacrum and Caudal Block

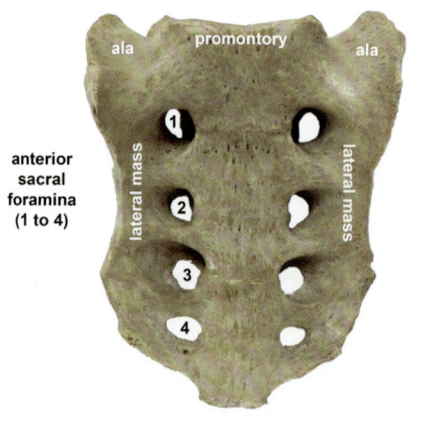

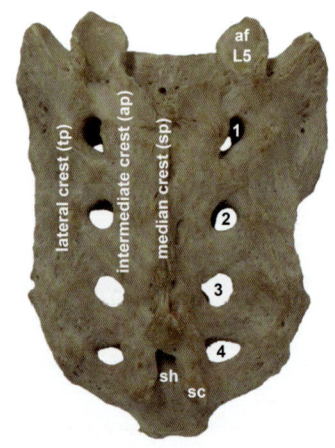

SOE2d Sacrum. Major features of sacrum. **af** articular facet; **ap** articular process; **sc** sacral cornu; **sh** sacral hiatus; **sp** spinous process; **tp** transverse process.

a) A six-month-old, otherwise well, boy is to undergo general anaesthesia for an inguinal hernia repair. What analgesic options would you consider?
Paracetamol
NSAID
Opiate (fentanyl under anaesthesia)
Local anaesthetic in wound
TAP/ilioinguinal nerve block
Caudal block

b) For what type of surgery may a caudal block provide adequate analgesia?
Most types of surgery of the abdomen/pelvis/genitalia/perineum below the umbilicus
General surgery: inguinal hernia repair, distal gastrointestinal tract (e.g. rectum/anus)
Urology: orchidopexy/orchidectomy, hypospadias repair, circumcision
(Sometimes lower limb plastic/orthopaedic surgery)

c) Describe the anatomy of the sacrum
Triangular bone at the bottom of the spine, formed by five fused sacral vertebrae
Wedged between hip bones, only the superior part is weight bearing (transmits weight of body to pelvic girdle)
Concave (more in males)

Base (uppermost, tilted anteriorly), apex and four surfaces (anterior, posterior and two lateral surfaces)
Central mass: formed by the fusion of five vertebral bodies
Laterally: two lateral masses (alae, wings), articulate with ilium at auricular surfaces (synovial joint)
Anterior surface:

- Sacral promontory
- Four transverse lines (represent fusion of vertebral bodies; complete after 20th year)
- Anterior sacral foramina

Dorsal surface:

- Median crest (fused spinous processes), medial/intermediate crest (fused articular processes) and lateral crest (fused transverse processes)
- Dorsal sacral foramina
- Sacral hiatus (absence of spine and failure of fusion of laminae of S5 +/− S4)
- Sacral cornua (articular processes of 5th sacral vertebra)
- Sacral hiatus closed by superficial sacrococcygeal ligament (sacrococcygeal membrane)

Sacral canal:

- Triangular, continuous with vertebral canal above, contains nerve roots of caudal equina
- Contains: termination of dural sac (sacral nerves and filum terminale), areolar connective tissue, venous plexus, lymphatics
- Filum terminale internum: dural sac attaches to back of S2 vertebra
- Filum terminale externum: continuation of pia attached to back of coccyx

d) **What are the anatomical considerations with regard to paediatric neuroaxial blockade?**
Spinal cord ends at L1/2 in adults, L3 in children
Dura ends at S2 in adults, S4 in children (adult level by age of 2 years)

e) **How can you identify the sacral hiatus?**
Apex of equilateral triangle completed by PSIS on each side
With hips flexed at 90°, longitudinal axis of femur points to sacral hiatus
Palpate the median (midline) sacral crest inferior until the cornua are identified

f) **What dose of 0.25% levo-bupivacaine would you use for this surgery?**
Armitage formula (1979) for 0.25% levo-bupivacaine:

- Sacral block: 0.5 ml/kg (circumcision, hypospadias, anal procedures)
- Low thoracic block: 1 ml/kg (hernia repair)
- Midthoracic (T8): 1.25 ml/kg (e.g. orchidopexy)

g) **What are the contraindications and complications of a caudal block?**
Contraindications:

- Lack of parental consent
- Lack of patient assent (older children)
- Local/systemic infection

- Coagulopathy
- Local anaesthetic allergy (or toxicity)
- Raised ICP
- CV instability (in children >6 years)

Complications:
- Failure
- Incorrect injection site: IV, IO, subdural/intrathecal, subcutaneous
- Drug reaction: local anaesthetic systemic toxicity, allergy to injected drugs
- Effects of local anaesthetic: motor block, urinary retention
- Epidural haematoma
- Bowel perforation
- Infection

Section 4 — SOEs 1–3 (Answers)

SOE 3a — Scalp Block

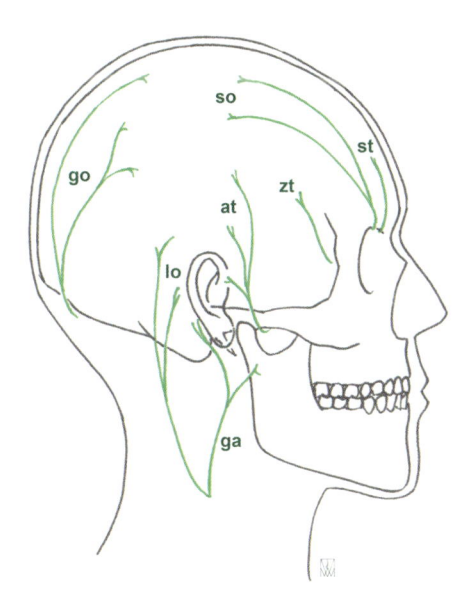

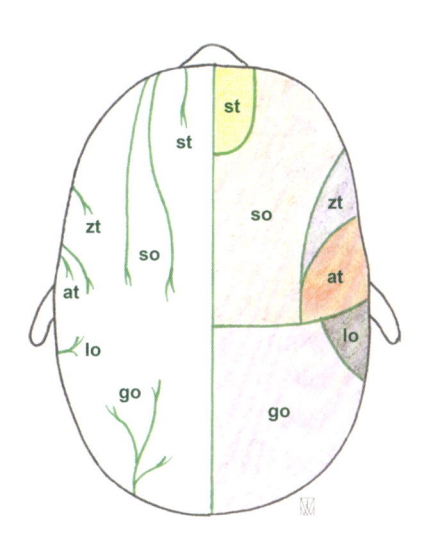

SOE3a Scalp. Cutaneous supply of scalp. Note that the greater occipital nerve is derived from dorsal rami. **at** auriculotemporal; **ga** great auricular; **go** greater occipital; **lo** lesser occipital; **so** supraorbital; **st** supratrochlear; **zt** zygomaticotemporal.

a) **On the image SOE3a, name the (seven pairs of) nerves targeted in a scalp block. Describe the region they supply.**

Supraorbital nerve:
- The larger branch of the frontal nerve (CN 5.1)
- Through supraorbital notch to supply forehead, upper eyelid and anterior scalp (to vertex)

Supratrochlear nerve:
- The smaller branch of the frontal nerve (CN 5.1)
- Innervates medial forehead, bridge of nose and medial portion of upper eyelid

Zygomaticotemporal nerve:
- Branch of the zygomatic nerve (CN 5.2)
- Passes through the zygomaticotemporal foramen of the zygoma, and then through temporalis muscle, to pierce the temporalis fascia

- Sensory innervation of lateral forehead and anterior temporal region ('hairless' part of temple)

Auriculotemporal nerve:
- Branch of CN 5.3
- Crosses zygomatic process of the temporal bone with the superficial temporal artery
- Innervates lateral surface of auricle, external auditory meatus, outer tympanic membrane and posterior temporal region ('hairy' part of temple)

Lesser occipital nerve:
- From *anterior ramus* of C2
- Ascends obliquely along the posterior border of sternocleidomastoid
- Provides sensory innervation to the scalp behind the auricle

Greater occipital nerve:
- Medial branch of the *posterior ramus* of C2
- Sensory innervation to the skin over the occiput and posterior scalp (up to the vertex), and posterior neck

Great auricular nerve (remember – no *greater* auricular nerve!)
- A branch of the (superficial/sensory) cervical plexus, with root values C2–3
- Emerges from behind the posterior border of sternocleidomastoid and travels directly up to supply the lateral surface of the auricle (below EAM) and all of its cranial surface, as well as skin over the parotid and angle of jaw

b) **Which of these nerves are derived from cranial nerves (and from which one)?**
Four of these nerves are derived from CN 5:
- Supraorbital nerve (from the frontal branch of CN 5.1)
- Supratrochlear nerve (from the frontal branch of CN 5.1)
- Zygomaticotemporal nerve (branch of zygomatic nerve, itself a branch of CN 5.2)
- Auriculotemporal nerve (branch of CN 5.3)

c) **What are the indications for a scalp block?**
Awake craniotomy
Postcraniotomy analgesia
Analgesia for scalp wound/suturing

d) **What landmarks are used to block each of these nerves as part of a scalp block?**
Supraorbital: supraorbital notch, inject immediately above periosteum
Supratrochlear: medial to supraorbital notch, inject immediately above periosteum (single midbrow skin insertion point can be used for bilateral blocks)
Zygomaticotemporal: from lateral edge of orbital margin along length of zygomatic arch, inject deep and superficial to temporalis muscle
Auriculotemporal: 1 cm anterior to the auricle (palpate superficial temporal artery to avoid accidental intra-arterial injection; nerve and artery lie together)
Lesser occipital: infiltrate at a point two-thirds of the way along a line from the external occipital protuberance to the mastoid process

SOE 3a: Scalp Block

Greater occipital: infiltrate at a point one-third of the way along a line from the external occipital protuberance to the mastoid process (greater occipital nerve runs with the occipital artery)

Great auricular: infiltrate 2 cm posterior to auricle, over the mastoid process, level with tragus

Section 4 — SOEs 1–3 (Answers)

SOE 3b — Fetal Circulation

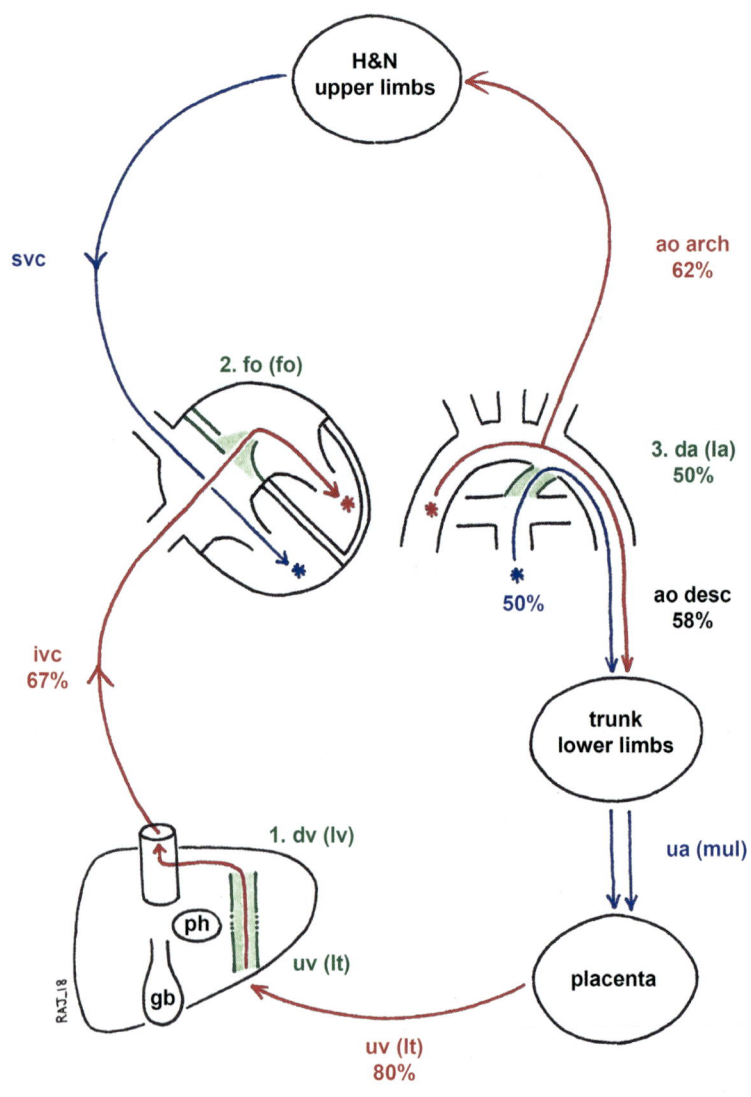

SOE3b Fetal circulation. Schematic. Note the three bypass mechanisms in the fetus (dv, fo, da) and the per cent oxygen saturation in the different parts of the circuit. **ao** aorta; **da (la)** ductus arteriosus (ligamentum arteriosum); **dv (lv)** ductus venosus (ligamentum venosum); **fo (fo)** foramen ovale (fossa ovalis); **gb** gall bladder; **ivc** inferior vena cava; **ph** porta hepatis; **svc** superior vena cava; **ua (mul)** umbilical artery (medial umbilical ligament); **uv (lt)** umbilical vein (ligamentum teres).

SOE 3b: Fetal Circulation

a) **Use the diagram SOE3b to describe the fetal circulation, starting at the umbilical vein**
   Oxygenated blood returns from the placenta via the (left) umbilical vein
   (The right umbilical vein obliterates during fetal development)
   This joins the left branch of the portal vein in the porta hepatis
   Most (>60%) travels to the IVC via the ductus venosus, bypassing the hepatic circulation
   On returning to the right atrium, oxygenated blood from the IVC travels across the foramen ovale to the left atrium
   From the left atrium blood passes to the left ventricle and out into the ascending aorta, perfusing the carotid arteries
   Deoxygenated blood returning from the head and neck via the SVC passes through the right atrium (mixing very little with oxygenated blood from the IVC) to the right ventricle, and out into the pulmonary trunk
   90% of this blood bypasses the lungs via the ductus arteriosus, which opens into the aorta distal to the three branches of the arch of the aorta (preventing venous blood from perfusing the head and neck)
   This deoxygenated blood then travels in the descending aorta and through the common iliac arteries, then (anterior division of the) internal iliac arteries, and finally the umbilical artery to the placenta

b) **Label the diagram with approximate oxygen saturation of blood at the following points:**
   Umbilical vein – 80%
   IVC – 67%
   Ascending aorta – 62%
   Ductus arteriosus – 50%
   Descending aorta – 58%

c) **What are the physiological changes that occur at birth?**
   When the neonate inspires, the expanding and newly oxygenated lung tissue causes a dramatic reduction in pulmonary vascular resistance
   As pulmonary blood flow increases, so does pulmonary venous return
   Clamping of the umbilical cord raises systemic vascular resistance and aortic pressure
   This raises left atrial pressure, causing closure of the foramen ovale
   As the pressure gradient across the left and right side of the circulation reverses, this reduces (or even reverses) blood flow across the ductus arteriosus
   The ductus arteriosus closes via contraction of its muscular wall due to higher partial pressures of oxygen and chemical mediators (e.g. decreasing prostaglandins)
   Obliteration of the ductus arteriosus can take from two weeks to two months

d) **Describe the development and structure of the foramen ovale***
   At early stages of embryonic development, a single atrium is present
   An initial partition grows down from the posterosuperior wall (septum primum) to meet the endocardial cushions, which divide the embryonic atria from ventricles
   Before the two atria are completely divided, a perforation develops in the septum primum, the foramen secundum (the foramen primum being the initial communication between the two sides of the atrium)
   A second partition then develops on the right of the septum primum (the septum secundum)

Section 4: SOEs 1–3 (Answers)

The septum secundum has a free lower border, but is large enough to overlap the foramen secundum

This creates a flap-valve effect:
- When the right atrium is at higher pressure, the septum primum deviates to the left, allowing blood to pass through the space between the foramen secundum and septum secundum (from right to left)
- However, when the left atrium is at higher pressure, the septum primum is compressed against the septum secundum, closing the channel

*This version is derived from a particularly excellent description in Ellis and Mahedevan's 'Clinical Anatomy: Applied Anatomy for Students and Junior Doctors' (12th Edition, 2010; pp. 40–4) – the authors encourage readers to review this account

e) **What is meant by a paradoxical embolus?**

This refers to an embolus that is carried from the venous side of the adult circulation to the arterial side (or vice versa)

It can cross via a defect in the heart, such as a patent foramen ovale (or ASD/VSD), or via AV shunts in the lungs

They represent around 2% of emboli

Section 4
SOE 3c

SOEs 1–3 (Answers)

Blood Supply of the Lower Limb and Intraosseous Access

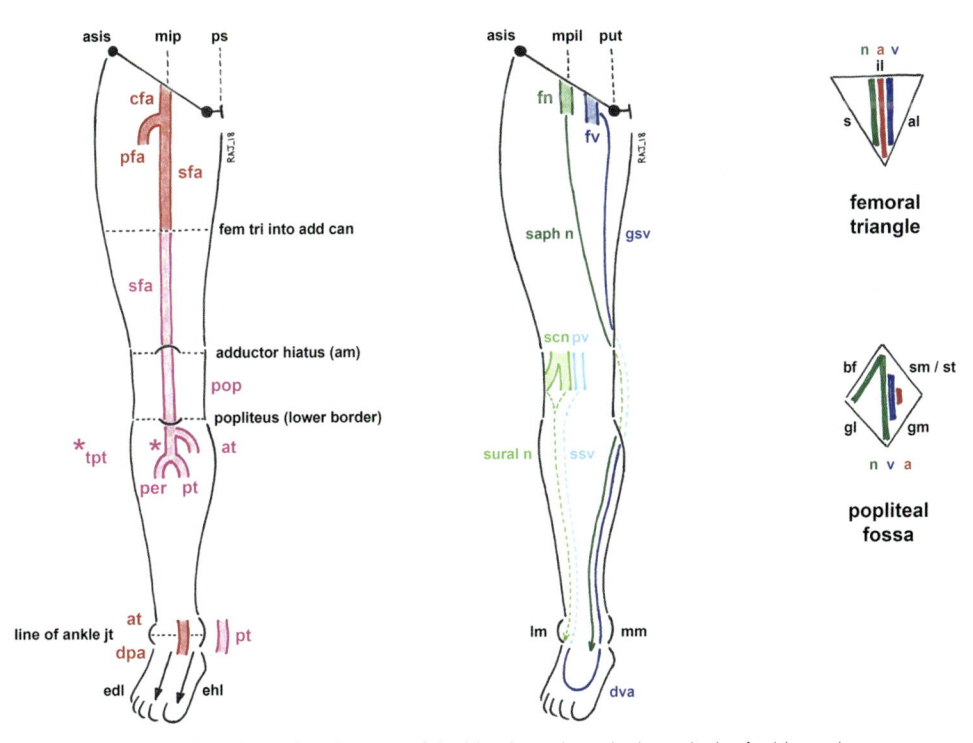

SOE3c Lower limb blood supply. Schematic of the blood supply to the lower limb. **al** adductor longus; **am** adductor magnus; **asis** anterior superior iliac spine; **at** anterior tibial artery; **bf** biceps femoris; **cfa** common femoral artery; **dp** deep peroneal nerve; **dpa** dorsalis pedis artery; **dva** dorsal venous arch; **edl** extensor digitorum longus; **ehl** extensor hallucis longus; **fn** femoral nerve; **fv** femoral vein; **gl** gastrocnemius lateral head; **gm** gastrocnemius medial head; **gsv** great saphenous vein; **il** inguinal ligament; **lm** lateral malleolus; **mip** midinguinal point; **mm** medial malleolus; **mpil** midpoint of inguinal ligament; **per** peroneal artery; **pfa** profunda femoris artery; **pop** popliteal artery; **ps** pubic symphysis; **pt** posterior tibial artery; **put** pubic tubercle; **pv** popliteal vein; **s** sartorius; **scn** sciatic nerve; **sfa** superficial femoral artery; **sm / st** semimembranosus/semitendinosus; **sn** saphenous nerve; **ssv** small saphenous vein; **t** tibial nerve; **tpt** tibioperoneal trunk.

a) **Describe the arterial supply of the lower limb**

The arterial supply is from the femoral artery, a continuation of the external iliac artery, entering the thigh under the inguinal ligament at the midinguinal point*

It initially lies in the lateral compartment of the femoral sheath, medial to the femoral nerve and lateral to the femoral vein

Section 4: SOEs 1–3 (Answers)

- Gives four small branches in the groin and courses distally in the femoral triangle, then in the adductor canal (under sartorius), lying on the anterior surface of muscles in the medial (adductor) compartment of the thigh
- In this course it gives off the profunda femoris (which passes posteriorly to supply the hip joint via circumflex branches and the posterior compartment of the thigh by perforating branches)
- It leaves the adductor canal by passing round the medial border of the femur (through the 'adductor hiatus' – defect in attachment of adductor magnus to the femur) and enters the popliteal fossa as the popliteal artery (where it gives branches to the knee joint)
- Divides at the lower border of popliteus into the posterior and anterior tibial arteries**
- The posterior tibial artery travels distally in the posterior compartment of the leg (calf); its most important branch is the peroneal artery (which supplies, but does not lie in, the lateral compartment of the leg)
- The posterior tibial artery passes behind the medial malleolus (where it is anterior to the tibial nerve), to enter the foot and divide into medial and lateral plantar arteries
- The anterior tibial artery travels in the anterior compartment of the leg and crosses the line of the ankle joint to become the dorsalis pedis artery

*Don't confuse these two locations:

- **Midinguinal point**: halfway between the ASIS and midline/pubic symphysis (where the femoral artery is found)
- **Midpoint of the inguinal ligament**: halfway between ASIS and the pubic tubercle (where the femoral nerve is found)

**Vascular surgeons/radiologists use slightly different terminology to anatomists and may refer to the above structures in these terms:

- **Common femoral artery** (CFA; from inguinal ligament to origin of profunda femoris)
- **Deep artery of the thigh** (profunda femoris)
- **Superficial femoral artery** (SFA; femoral artery from origin of profunda femoris to adductor hiatus)
- **Tibioperoneal trunk** (TPT; the short segment of the posterior tibial artery, before the peroneal artery arises)

b) **Describe the course of the great/long saphenous vein**
   Begins as a continuation of the dorsal venous arch, on the medial side of the dorsum of the foot
   Lies *in front* of the medial malleolus and courses proximally, following an oblique course across the superficial surface of the distal tibia (from anterior to posterior)
   Passes a hand's breadth *behind* the medial border of the patella, then courses up the anteromedial thigh to enter the femoral vein at the saphenous opening

c) **Name the principal superficial vein on the posterior surface of the leg**
   Small/short saphenous vein

SOE 3c: Blood Supply of the Lower Limb and Intraosseous Access

d) **With which nerves do these two veins run in the leg?**
   Great/long saphenous vein: saphenous nerve (from the femoral nerve)
   Small/short saphenous vein: sural nerve (from the tibial and common peroneal nerves)

e) **Name two sites for intraosseous vascular access in the lower limb**
   Proximal tibia (2 cm medial and 2 cm below the tibial tuberosity, on the medial/subcutaneous surface)
   Distal tibia (around 3 cm proximal to the medial malleolus, on the medial/subcutaneous surface)
   Distal femur (around 3 cm above and 2 cm medial to the lateral epicondyle)

f) **Name the indications and contraindications to intraosseous access**
   Indications:
   - Any clinical situation requiring blood sampling or vascular access (but this is not immediately possible)
   - Inability to gain vascular access in emergency management where intravascular access/drugs/fluids are required (e.g. trauma, shock)
   - During CPR (particularly in children)

   Contraindications:
   - Site of bone fracture
   - Ipsilateral fracture of the extremity (particularly in the same bone)
   - Difficulty identifying anatomy
   - Infection (or burn) at site of entry
   - Site of previous attempt/access within 48 hours (or different sites on same bone)
   - Compartment syndrome in same limb
   - Site of prosthesis

| Section 4 | SOEs 1–3 (Answers) |

SOE 3d Orbit

a.

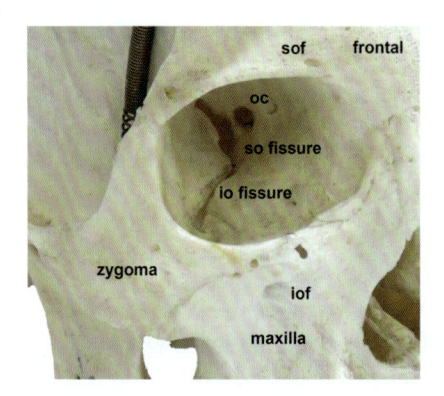

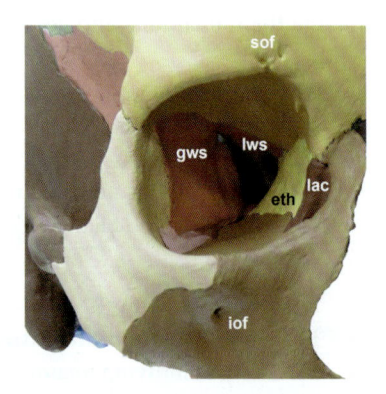

b.

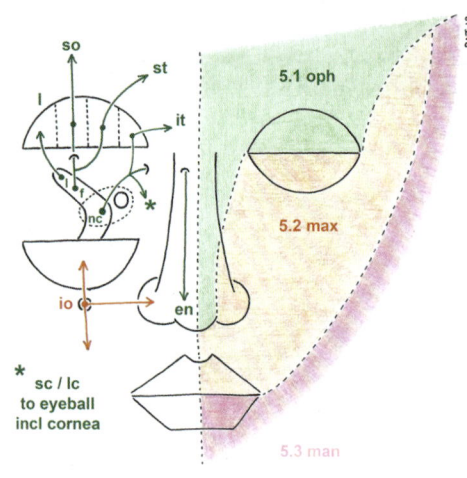

c.

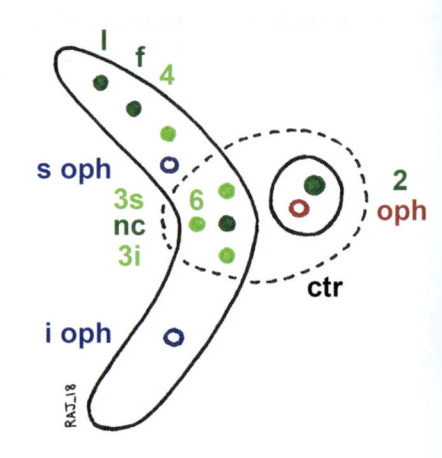

SOE3d Orbit. a. Bony features of orbit. b. Schematic – course of sensory nerves of orbit. c. Schematic – optic canal and orbital fissures. Note structures passing within and outside common tendinous ring. **3i** oculomotor inferior division; **3s** oculomotor superior division; **ctr** common tendinous ring; **en** external nasal; **eth** ethmoid; **f** frontal; **gws** greater wing of sphenoid; **i oph** inferior ophthalmic vein; **io** infraorbital; **io fissure** inferior orbital fissure; **iof** infraorbital foramen; **it** infratrochlear; **l** lacrimal; **lac** lacrimal; **lws** lesser wing of sphenoid; **man** mandibular; **max** maxillary; **nc** nasociliary; **oc** optic canal; **oph** ophthalmic artery; **s oph** superior ophthalmic vein; **sc / lc** short ciliary/long ciliary; **so** supraorbital; **so fissure** superior orbital fissure; **sof** supraorbital foramen; **st** supratrochlear.

a) **Describe the bony structure of the orbit**

Four-sided pyramid, lying on its side

The base lies anteriorly and apex posteriorly (on the optic canal/medial end of the superior orbital fissure)

Medial walls lie in parallel and lateral walls diverge at 90° (continuing these lines posteriorly, they would meet at the pituitary fossa)*

Roof:
- Orbital plate of frontal bone
- Lesser wing of sphenoid

Floor:
- Orbital surface of maxilla
- Partly by zygomatic and palatine bones

Medial wall:
- Orbit plate of ethmoid bone (lamina papyracea)
- Contributions from the maxilla, lacrimal and sphenoid

Lateral wall (longest, thickest and strongest part of the orbit):
- Zygomatic bone
- Greater wing of sphenoid

*Note that the axes of the orbit and globe are different:
- The axis of the orbit bisects the medial and lateral walls, i.e. lies along a plane that runs from posteromedial to anterolateral
- The axis of the globe lies on a direct anteroposterior plane

b) **On this image of the orbit, identify features A–E**
   A) Optic canal
   B) Superior orbital fissure
   C) Inferior orbital fissure
   D) Supraorbital foramen (more commonly the foramen is not complete, when it is termed the supraorbital notch)
   E) Infraorbital groove, canal and foramen

c) **Which areas do A and B run between, and what structures do they transmit?**
   A) Optic canal:
   - Canal through the lesser wing of the sphenoid bone
   - Connects orbit to middle cranial fossa
   - Transmits CN 2 and the ophthalmic artery

   B) Superior orbital fissure:
   - Cleft between greater and lesser wings of sphenoid
   - Connects orbit and middle cranial fossa
   - Divided into three compartments by the common tendinous origin/ring (annulus of Zinn), which gives rise to rectus muscles in the orbit

- Lateral compartment: lacrimal (CN 5.1), frontal (CN 5.1) and trochlear (CN 4) nerves, superior ophthalmic vein
- Intermediate compartment (within the tendinous ring): oculomotor (CN 3; superior and inferior divisions), abducens (CN 6) and nasociliary (CN 5.1) nerves
- Medial compartment: inferior ophthalmic vein

d) **What is the nerve supply to the eye?**

Sensory:
- CN 2 (vision)
- CN 5.1 (general sensation, via long and short ciliary nerves, which come from nasociliary nerves)

Sympathetic:
- T1 fibres that synapse in the superior cervical ganglion
- Travel superiorly in the neck in the carotid plexus
- Join CN 5.1 in the cavernous sinus
- Pass forwards through the superior orbital fissure on the nasociliary nerve, then the long ciliary nerves
- Stimulation leads to contraction of the radial muscles of the iris (dilator pupillae) causing pupil dilation

Parasympathetic:
- From the Edinger Westphal nucleus accompanying CN 3 (inferior division)
- Synapse in the ciliary ganglion, then run in the short ciliary nerves
- Stimulation leads to contraction of the ciliary muscle (lens accommodation) and the sphincter pupillae muscle (pupil constriction)

e) **What blocks are used to provide anaesthesia in surgery on the eye?**

Topical administration of local anaesthesia

Peribulbar block (outwith cone of muscles that surround the globe: the muscles have a thin fibrous layer running between them, so larger volumes (5–15 ml) of local anaesthetic are administered, which diffuses into the cone to contact the nerves)

Retrobulbar block (outwith Tenon's capsule of the globe but within the surrounding cone of muscles/fascia, therefore smaller volumes (3–5 ml) of local anaesthetic needed)

Sub-Tenon's block (injection of local anaesthetic under the capsule of the eye, which is continuous with the cuff of dura around the optic nerve)

Section 5 MCQs 1–60 (Answers)

T = true; F = false

1. **The anterior triangle of the neck:**
   Is bounded posteriorly by the anterior border of sternocleidomastoid [T]
   Contains the carotid sheath [T]
   Contains the external jugular vein [F]
   Is overlain by skin supplied by the transverse cervical nerve(s) [T]
   Is bounded superiorly by the lower border of the mandible [T]

The anterior triangle of the neck contains the *internal* jugular vein, not the external jugular vein.

2. **Regarding the anterolateral abdominal wall:**
   The lumbar triangle (of Petit) is bounded by the posterior border of the external oblique muscle, the anterior border of the latissimus dorsi muscle and the iliac crest [T]
   The floor of the lumbar triangle (of Petit) is formed by the transversus abdominis muscle [F]
   During a landmark technique TAP block, two 'pops' are felt as the needle passes through the thoracolumbar fascia and external oblique layer [F]
   A subcostal TAP block can be used for surgery extending above the umbilicus [T]
   The external oblique, internal oblique and transversus abdominis muscles all have the same innervation, which is solely from the thoracoabdominal (T7–11) and subcostal (T12) nerves [F]

The floor of the inferior lumbar triangle (of Petit) is formed by internal oblique muscle. The two 'pops' felt during a TAP block are from the needle passing through the aponeuroses of the external then internal oblique muscles. The internal oblique and transversus abdominis muscles are also supplied by the iliohypogastric and ilioinguinal nerves (L1).

3. **At the ankle:**
   All of the deep nerves supplying the foot are branches of the sciatic nerve [T]
   The deep peroneal nerve enters the dorsum of the foot between the tendons of extensor hallucis longus and extensor digitorum longus [T]
   The deep peroneal nerve is a hyperechoic structure on ultrasound [T]
   The superficial peroneal nerve emerges between extensor digitorum longus and peroneus brevis [T]
   The sural nerve lies anterior to the medial malleolus [F]

The saphenous nerve is a branch of the femoral nerve. The sural nerve lies posterior to the lateral malleolus and is associated with the short saphenous vein.

4. Regarding the larynx and trachea:
    In the adult, the narrowest part of the upper respiratory tract is at the level of the cricoid cartilage [F]
    In the child, the narrowest part of the upper respiratory tract is at the level of the (open) vocal cords [F]
    The position of the carina moves with respiration [T]
    The trachea is in contact with the left vagus nerve in the thorax [F]
    The trachea is in contact with the thoracic duct posteriorly [F]

The cricoid cartilage is the narrowest part of the upper respiratory tract in the child, in the adult it is at the vocal cords. The left vagus nerve lies on the arch of the aorta (not the trachea) and the thoracic duct lies behind and in contact with the oesophagus (not the trachea).

5. The following is true of the ribs:
    The sympathetic trunk is an anterior relation of the neck of the first rib [T]
    Typical ribs have a head with two articular facets, for articulation with their own vertebra and the one below [F]
    Typical ribs have a tubercle with a smooth articular facet, which forms a synovial joint with the transverse process of the corresponding vertebra [T]
    Typical ribs have a tubercle with a rough non-articular facet, for attachment of the lateral costotransverse ligament [T]
    The costal cartilages of ribs 2–10 form primary cartilaginous joints with the sternum or rib/costal cartilage above [F]

More specifically, the stellate/cervicothoracic ganglion lies on the anterior surface of the neck of the first rib. Typical ribs do have two articular facets, but they articulate with the corresponding vertebra and the one above. The costal cartilages of ribs 2–10 form a synovial joint with the sternum or costal cartilage above.

6. Regarding autonomic dysreflexia:
    Excess sympathetic discharge occurs in response to stimuli below level of spinal cord lesion [T]
    Features are more pronounced with higher lesions and a stronger reaction is observed if a more proximal dermatome is stimulated [F]
    Patients develop tachycardia/arrhythmias, with severe hypotension and headache [F]
    Below the level of the spinal cord lesion, patients exhibit sweating, pallor and muscle contraction/spasticity [T]
    Central neuroaxial blockade can be used to prevent and manage autonomic dysreflexia [T]

After a transecting injury of the spinal cord, stimulation of spinal cord reflexes below the level of the injury are exaggerated due to the loss of descending inhibition from higher centres. Features are more pronounced with stimulation of more distal/lower levels. Patients typically develop severe hypertension with reflex bradycardia.

7. The following are true of the internal auditory meatus/auditory canal:
    It transmits the vestibulocochlear nerve and the facial nerve [T]
    It is directed laterally in the petrous bone [T]
    It connects the middle cranial fossa to the inner ear [F]
    It contains only the motor component of CN 7 [F]
    The vestibular ganglion lies within the internal auditory meatus [T]

The internal auditory meatus/auditory canal connects the *posterior* cranial fossa and inner ear. The vestibular ganglion (equivalent to the DRG of a spinal nerve) lies within the IAM.

8. Regarding the rectus abdominis:
   The rectus abdominis muscle lies superficial to the external oblique aponeurosis [F]
   The superior epigastric artery is a branch of the internal thoracic artery [T]
   The arcuate line of the rectus sheath lies approximately halfway between the pubic symphysis and umbilicus [T]
   Motor supply of the rectus abdominis is partly by the iliohypogastric nerve [F]
   Perforation of the inferior epigastric artery is a common complication of rectus sheath block [F]

The external oblique aponeurosis contributes to the anterior layer of the rectus sheath, hence the rectus abdominis muscle lies deep to it. Motor supply to rectus abdominis is from the thoracoabdominal (T7–11) and subcostal (T12) nerves. Perforation of the inferior epigastric artery is a minor risk of rectus sheath block, especially when performed at or below the level of the umbilicus.

9. The following is true of the lower limb vasculature:
   The femoral artery lies in the adductor (subsartorial/Hunter's) canal [T]
   The inferior epigastric artery is a branch of the femoral artery [F]
   The femoral vein lies medial to the femoral artery initially, but lies posteriorly to it at the apex of the femoral triangle [T]
   The popliteal vein is the deepest structure in the popliteal fossa [F]
   The peroneal artery provides little or no arterial supply to the foot [T]

The inferior epigastric artery arises from the external iliac artery, just before the latter passes beneath the inguinal ligament to become the femoral artery. The popliteal artery is the deepest structure in the popliteal fossa, making it difficult to palpate. The peroneal (fibular) artery arises from the tibioperoneal trunk, along with the posterior tibial artery, and supplies the lateral compartment of the leg. The foot is supplied by the anterior and posterior tibial arteries, the former becoming the dorsalis pedis artery as it crosses the ankle joint into the foot.

10. Regarding the scalp block:
    The infraorbital nerve is targeted [F]
    The transverse cervical nerves are targeted [F]
    The third occipital nerve is targeted [F]
    A scalp block can be the sole technique used for awake craniotomy, without sedation or general anaesthesia, as the brain itself is not sensitive to painful stimuli [T]
    Intra-arterial injection into the superficial temporal artery is possible when targeting the auriculotemporal nerve [T]

The *supraorbital* (not infraorbital) nerve is targeted (although the infratrochlear nerve may be affected due to its proximity). The greater and lesser occipital nerves are targeted, whilst the third occipital usually supplies posterior skin further down the neck. However, since the greater and third occipital nerves often communicate (being derived from the dorsal rami of C2 and C3, respectively), the spread of local anaesthetic may

inadvertently block the third occipital nerve. The auriculotemporal nerve travels with the superficial temporal artery, which can be damaged (or injected) when performing a scalp block.

11. Regarding the lungs and pleura:
    The pulmonary ligament consists of pleura [T]
    The visceral pleura has no sensory innervation [F]
    At the midpoint between full inspiration and expiration, the inferior border of the lung lies at the level of the sixth rib in the midclavicular line [T]
    The horizontal fissure of the right lung lies at the level of the fourth costal cartilage and runs horizontally backwards to meet the oblique fissure in the midaxillary line [T]
    The blunt posterior border of the lung lies in the paravertebral gutter, either side of the midline [T]

The pulmonary ligament is a fold/cuff of pleura at the lung root, formed by the reflection/continuity of the parietal and visceral layers, which provides dead space for lung root to descend during inspiration and permits expansion of the pulmonary vessels. The visceral pleura receives nociceptive innervation via sympathetic nerves of the pulmonary plexus (which enter/leave the lung via the root). The inferior border of the lung lies behind the 6th rib in the midclavicular line, 8th rib in midaxillary line, 10th rib in midscapular line (lateral border of erector spinae) and from there passes horizontally to the lower border of the T10 vertebra. The oblique fissure of both lungs starts posteriorly at the level of the spinous process of T3, then runs downwards and forwards to lie behind the 6th rib in the midclavicular line (roughly in line with the 5th rib). The sharp anterior and inferior borders lie in the costomediastinal and costodiaphragmatic recesses respectively.

12. Regarding Brown–Séquard syndrome:
    It typically results after complete transection of the spinal cord [F]
    It results in an ipsilateral upper motor neurone lesion (spastic paralysis) below the level of the injury [T]
    It results in an ipsilateral lower motor neurone lesion (flaccid paralysis) below the level of the injury [F]
    It results in ipsilateral loss of vibration sensation and proprioception (dorsal column) below the level of the injury [T]
    It results in contralateral loss of pain and temperature sensation (spinothalamic tract) below the level of the injury [T]

Brown–Séquard syndrome follows hemisection of the spinal cord, resulting in a lower motor neurone lesion at the level of the injury (damage to the anterior grey horn). However, the injury also transects the white matter columns:
   Descending fibres of the corticospinal tract (upper motor neurones, which have already decussated proximally)
   Ascending fibres of the spinothalamic tract (second order sensory neurones, which decussated at the level of entry of the first order sensory neurone in the peripheral spinal nerve)

Ascending fibres of the dorsal column–medial lemniscal pathway (first order neurones, which are destined to synapse and then decussate more proximally)

This leads to paralysis and loss of vibration/proprioception below the level of the injury on the same side of the body, but loss of pain/temperature sensation on the opposite side.

13. The following bones contribute to the pterion:
    Sphenoid (greater wing) [T]
    Frontal [T]
    Temporal (squamous part) [T]
    Parietal [T]
    Occipital [F]

14. Regarding the bronchial circulation:
    The bronchial arteries supply the lung parenchyma with oxygenated blood [T]
    The bronchial arteries arise from the corresponding pulmonary artery [F]
    There are two bronchial arteries supplying the right lung [F]
    The bronchial veins return deoxygenated blood directly to the inferior vena cava [F]
    The bronchial and pulmonary circulations allow mixing of oxygenated and deoxygenated blood [T]

Two bronchial arteries arise from the descending thoracic aorta to supply the left lung, the single bronchial artery to the right lung arises from the third right posterior intercostal artery. The superficial bronchial veins drain the surface of the lung to the azygos system of veins; the deep bronchial veins drain the deeper tissue to either the pulmonary veins or directly into the left atrium (and this contributes to the mixing of oxygenated and deoxygenated blood; known as shunt*).

*N.B. The venae cordis minimae of the heart also contribute to shunt, as some of the venules also drain directly into the left atrium

15. Regarding the blood supply of the upper limb:
    The axillary artery is a continuation of the subclavian artery at the lateral border of scalenus anterior [F]
    The cords of the brachial plexus are named according to their relationship to the second part of the axillary artery [T]
    The axillary artery gives rise to medial and lateral circumflex humeral arteries [F]
    The ulnar artery gives rise to the common interosseous artery [T]
    The superficial (palmar) branch of the radial artery travels into the hand deep to the flexor retinaculum [F]

The subclavian artery becomes the axillary artery at the outer border of first rib. The second part of the axillary artery lies behind pectoralis minor, surrounded by the cords of the brachial plexus. The axillary artery gives rise to the *anterior/posterior* circumflex humeral arteries (the femoral artery gives rise to *medial/lateral* circumflex femoral arteries). The common interosseous artery divides into anterior and posterior interosseous arteries, which travel with anterior (from the median) and posterior (from the radial) nerves respectively. The superficial (palmar) branch of the radial artery lies superficial to the flexor retinaculum.

16. **The following is true regarding relations of the orbit:**
    The anterior cranial fossa is a superior relation of the orbit [T]
    The ethmoid air sinuses are a medial relation of the orbit [T]
    The sphenoid air sinus is a posterior relation of the orbit [F]
    The maxillary air sinus is a medial relation of the orbit [F]
    The infratemporal fossa and middle cranial fossa are posterolateral relations of the orbit [T]

The anterior cranial fossa and frontal lobe lie above the orbit. The ethmoid sinuses and upper part of the nasal cavity lie between the orbits. The maxillary air sinus lies below the orbit. The sphenoidal sinus lies between the posterior extent of the orbits.

17. **Which of the following are boundaries of the paravertebral space?**
    The superior costotransverse ligament is a superior boundary [F]
    The visceral pleura of the thorax is an anterolateral boundary [F]
    The psoas muscle is an anterolateral boundary at the lumbar level [T]
    The endothoracic fascia is a medial boundary [F]
    The vertebral body is a medial boundary [T]

The superior costotransverse ligament is a *posterior* boundary and the *parietal* pleura is an anterolateral boundary. The endothoracic fascia is found between the parietal pleura and the ribs/innermost layer of intercostal muscles.

18. **Regarding central cord syndrome:**
    It is commonly due to a crush injury (without transection) of the spinal cord [T]
    Hyperextension of the cervical spine is a common feature [T]
    The upper limbs are affected more than the lower limbs [T]
    The cervical fibres of the spinothalamic tract are more superficial than the sacral fibres [F]
    The anterior horn of grey matter is not affected [F]

Since the cell bodies of the lower motor neurones to the upper limb muscles are located more centrally in the anterior grey horn, the upper limbs are preferentially affected in central cord syndrome.

19. **Regarding sutures of the cranium:**
    They are secondary cartilaginous joints [F]
    They fuse at around 20–40 years of age [T]
    The lambda represents the closed/ossified posterior fontanelle [T]
    The anterior fontanelle closes/ossifies after the posterior fontanelle [T]
    An extradural haematoma crosses lines of sutural intersection [T]

The sutures of the cranium are fibrous joints. The sutures fuse between ages 20 and 40 years, from the inside to out. Initially, the sutural joints provide mobility required during parturition and then growth of the brain. The lambda represents the closed/ossified posterior fontanelle – the point of intersection between the sagittal (between parietal bones) and lambdoid (between parietal and occipital bones) sutures. Closure occurs in the first year and can be as early as 6–8 weeks. The larger anterior fontanelle closes at around 12–18 months to form the bregma – the point of intersection between the coronal and sagittal sutures. An extradural haematoma can cross lines of sutural intersection since it develops between the dura mater and the endocranium* (periosteum of bone on the inner surface of the cranium). In comparison, a fracture-haematoma is limited by periosteal boundaries as the periosteum of bone on inner and outer surfaces of the cranium is fused with the sutural joint. This type of haematoma is therefore limited by sutural joints to the margins of the involved bone.

*N.B. The endocranium is sometimes, confusingly, referred to as the 'outer layer of dura', with the dura mater proper then referred to as 'inner layer of dura'.

20. **The following is true in relation to the right lung root:**
    The right upper lobe bronchus and accompanying artery are found above the main bronchus [T]
    The pulmonary arteries lie anterior to their respective bronchi [T]
    Four pulmonary veins drain the lung [F]
    Branches of the phrenic nerve supply the lung parenchyma [F]
    Pulmonary lymphatics drain the lung via this route [T]

The eparterial bronchus (to the right upper lobe) branches off before the right main bronchus reaches the hilum of the lung. Each lung drains by two pulmonary veins to the left atrium. The lung parenchyma receives an autonomic supply; the parietal pleura receives a somatic innervation from the intercostal (T1–6), thoracoabdominal (T7–11), subcostal and phrenic nerves. Branches of the pulmonary plexus (autonomic) pass through the hilum of the lung to innervate the lung parenchyma.

21. **Regarding the brachial plexus:**
    It comprises five roots, three trunks, five divisions and three cords [F]
    The branching pattern of the brachial plexus often varies between the right and left sides in the same individual [T]
    The sheath surrounding the brachial plexus is at its smallest volume in the supraclavicular fossa [T]
    The roots lie anterior to the anterior scalene muscle [F]
    It provides motor innervation to the serratus anterior muscle [T]

Each trunk of the brachial plexus gives anterior and posterior divisions (i.e. six in total). The roots emerge between scalenus anterior (in front) and medius (behind). (N.B. The posterior scalene muscle is part of the middle scalene, which continues down to attach to the second rib.) The long thoracic nerve (C5/6/7), arising from the roots of the brachial plexus, provides the motor innervation to serratus anterior (and therefore brachial plexus injury can lead to winging of the scapula).

22. **The following bones contribute to the orbital margin/rim:**
    Frontal [T]
    Zygomatic [T]
    Maxilla [T]
    Nasal [F]
    Ethmoid [F]

The frontal, zygomatic bone and maxilla contribute approximately one-third each to the orbital rim. The ethmoid contributes to the medial wall of the orbit, the nasal bone to the bridge of the nose.

23. Concerning the oesophageal sphincters:
    Atropine reduces lower oesophageal sphincter pressure [T]
    The lower oesophageal sphincter is in a state of tonic contraction [T]
    The upper oesophagus consists of skeletal muscle, but is not under voluntary control [T]
    Upper oesophageal sphincter tone is reduced by all intravenous anaesthetic induction agents [F]
    Upper oesophageal sphincter tone is reduced by both non-depolarising and depolarising neuromuscular blocking drugs [T]

Upper oesophageal sphincter tone is not reduced by ketamine.

24. Regarding anterior spinal artery syndrome:
    Proprioception is preserved below the level of the lesion [T]
    Voluntary motor function is lost below the level of the lesion [T]
    An upper motor neurone lesion (spastic paralysis) will develop below the level of the lesion [T]
    Pain and temperature sensation is preserved below the level of the lesion [F]
    The lateral spinothalamic tract is typically affected [T]

Anterior spinal artery syndrome causes ischaemia/infarction of the anterior two-thirds of the cord (and medulla), affecting the spinothalamic (pain/temperature) corticospinal (motor) tracts. A lower motor neurone lesion is seen *at the level of the lesion* and an upper motor neurone lesion below. Vibration sense and proprioception is conveyed in the dorsal column-medial lemniscal pathway, which is preserved.

25. The carotid sheath:
    Contains the external carotid artery [F]
    Contains the internal jugular vein [T]
    Contains the recurrent laryngeal nerve [F]
    Contains the ansa cervicalis within its anterior wall [T]
    Lies anterior to the phrenic nerve [T]

The carotid sheath contains the *common* carotid artery inferiorly and the *internal* carotid artery superiorly (after it bifurcates at the level of C4/upper border of the thyroid cartilage). The external carotid artery leaves the sheath to supply structures of the face and facial skeleton. The sheath also contains CN 10 (but not its recurrent laryngeal branch, which runs in the tracheo-oesophageal groove).

N.B. A note on the carotid sheath – unlike the investing fascia of the neck, the carotid sheath is not a separate entity/distinct fascial layer per se:
- Anterior wall is a thickening of posterior layer of deep investing fascia of the neck
- Medial wall is a thickening of the lateral wall of the pretracheal fascia
- Posterior wall is a thickening of the anterior wall of the prevertebral fascia

26. Regarding the coronary circulation:
    There are no anastomoses between the regions of arterial supply in the heart [F]
    80–90% of coronary venous circulation is returned to the right atrium via the coronary sinus [T]
    Blood supply to the right ventricle ceases during systole [F]
    The myocardium typically extracts approximately 50% of oxygen from arterial blood [T]
    The right ventricle is mainly supplied by the right coronary artery, originating from the proximal pulmonary trunk [F]

Anastomoses exist at the arteriolar level, 'potential anastomoses', which can develop a collateral circulation in chronic ischaemic heart disease (but are unable to prevent ischaemia in the event of an acute atheromatous plaque rupture during myocardial infarction). Arterial blood to the *left* ventricle ceases during systole, but the right (lower pressure) ventricle is supplied by arterial blood (at higher/systemic pressure) throughout the cardiac cycle. The right coronary artery arises from the proximal ascending aorta.

27. Regarding the brachial plexus:
    The divisions lie in the infraclavicular fossa [F]
    The trunks lie anterior to the subclavian artery [F]
    The three cords are described in relation to the subclavian artery [F]
    Pectoralis major lies anterior to the cords [T]
    The supraclavicular nerve typically branches from the upper trunk [T]

The divisions lie behind (or slightly above) the clavicle and the trunks lie posterior to the subclavian artery*. The three cords are described/named in relation to the second part of the axillary artery (the continuation of the subclavian artery at the outer border of the first rib).

> *Remember the heart lies anterior to the spinal cord, hence the nerves originate from a more posterior position than the vessels

28. CN 3 (the oculomotor nerve) supplies the following muscles of the orbit/eye:
    Lateral rectus [F]
    Superior oblique [F]
    Levator palpebrae superioris [T]
    Medial rectus [T]
    Dilator muscle of the iris [F]

A helpful aide-memoire for the nerve supply of muscles in the orbit is the 'formula' LR_6SO_4*. The lateral rectus is supplied by CN 6, superior oblique by CN 4, and all others by CN 3. The superior division of CN 3 supplies superior rectus and levator palpebrae superioris (which also has sympathetic innervation). The inferior division of CN 3 supplies medial rectus, inferior rectus and inferior oblique. The constrictor muscle of the iris is innervated by parasympathetic fibres of CN 3; the dilator muscle is supplied by the long ciliary nerves, carrying sympathetic fibres that have hitch-hiked along the nasociliary nerve (CN 5.1).

*As described in *Last's Anatomy: Regional and Applied*, by C Sinnatamby (12th Edition, 2011; p.401)

29. **Regarding oesophageal pathology:**
    Boerhaave's syndrome refers to oesophageal rupture secondary to iatrogenic injury [F]
    Nasogastric tube placement is contraindicated in the presence of oesophageal varices [F]
    Achalasia refers to failure of the lower oesophageal sphincter to relax [T]
    Adenocarcinoma of the oesophagus occurs mainly in the distal third [T]
    Approximately 80% of oesophageal cancer occurs in men [T]

Boerhaave's syndrome refers to oesophageal rupture associated with vomiting. Concern over variceal bleeding provoked by blind nasogastric tube placement in patients with known varices originated from expert opinion, but this has not been substantiated by published evidence to date. Equally, rebleeding frequency and transfusion rate has not been shown to be different with or without nasogastric tube insertion following ruptured oesophageal varices. There are clear benefits to the use of nasogastric tubes in critically unwell patients, and these must be weighed against the perceived risk of precipitating bleeding by insertion.

30. **The following is true with regard to adult and paediatric neuroaxial blockade:**
    The spinal cord ends at L1/2 in adults, but lower in children [T]
    The dura ends at S2 in adults, but higher in children [F]
    The subarachnoid space extends into the sacral canal [T]
    The male sacrum displays a greater curvature than the female sacrum [T]
    The sacrum articulates with four bones [T]

In children, the spinal cord ends at L3 and the dura at S4 (but reaches the adult level of S2 by the age of 2 years). Since the dural sac extends to S2, the subarachnoid space also extends to S2 and can therefore be entered via the sacral canal. Sex differences of the sacrum are pronounced, with the shape of the female sacrum adapted for parturition (shorter, wider and less curved). The sacrum articulates with the L5 vertebra, the coccyx and the ilium on either side.

31. **The following is true of the muscular branches of the cervical plexus (aka deep cervical plexus):**
    The phrenic nerve (C3/4/5) is not a branch of the cervical plexus [F]
    The parietal pleura receives sensory innervation from a muscular branch of the cervical plexus [T]
    The ansa cervicalis (C1–3) forms part of this plexus [T]
    Branches from C2/3 and C3/4 transmit proprioceptive sensation from sternocleidomastoid and trapezius [T]
    The cervical plexus does not innervate any structures inside the cranial cavity [F]

The phrenic nerve is a branch of the deep cervical plexus and provides the sole motor supply of the diaphragm. It also provides sensory innervation to the central diaphragm, mediastinal and (central part of the) diaphragmatic parietal pleura, fibrous/parietal pericardium and (central part of the) diaphragmatic parietal peritoneum. Meningeal

branches (C1–3) provide sensory supply to the dura and arachnoid mater in posterior cranial fossa.

> N.B. Ansa cervicalis
> - Superior root (C1): formed from hitch-hiking fibres of C1 that peel off from CN 12 (distal to the branches to geniohyoid and thyrohyoid); after leaving CN 12, the superior root travels down in the anterior wall of the carotid sheath to meet the inferior root
> - Inferior root (C2/3): forms behind the IJV, travels down in the carotid sheath and courses around the lateral side of the IJV to meet the superior root
> - Supplies three of the four strap muscles: sternothyroid, sternohyoid and omohyoid (thyrohyoid is supplied from the hitch-hiking fibres of C1 travelling with CN 12)

32. Regarding the diaphragm:
The central part is derived from the pleuroperitoneal membranes [F]
The central tendon is derived from the septum transversum [T]
It arises in part from the lateral arcuate ligament [T]
The sympathetic chain enters the abdomen behind the medial arcuate ligament [T]
The median arcuate ligament forms the aortic hiatus [T]

The peripheral part of the diaphragm is largely derived from the pleuroperitoneal membranes (with a contribution from the body wall); the central part is largely from the septum transversum, a fibrous division that lies between the heart and abdominal structures during development (with a contribution from the dorsal oesophageal mesentery).

> See OSCE Station 8 (Diaphragm) figure for information on other structures passing through/behind the diaphragm
>
> N.B. The arcuate ligaments:
>
> Median: formed by fibres from the medial parts of the right and left crura of the diaphragm
> Medial: a thickening of psoas fascia over the psoas muscle, running from the body of T2 (left) or T3 (right) to the transverse process of T1
> Lateral: a thickening of psoas fascia over the quadratus lumborum muscle, running from the transverse process of T1 to the 12th rib

33. Regarding the axillary brachial plexus block:
It reliably blocks the intercostobrachial nerve [F]
Motor innervation to biceps brachii is via the musculocutaneous nerve [T]
The axillary artery typically lies posterior to the conjoint tendon of teres major and latissimus dorsi [F]
The musculocutaneous nerve appears as a hypoechoic structure, due to the lack of connective tissue [F]
The axillary nerve is normally blocked [F]

The intercostobrachial nerve is the lateral cutaneous branch of the second intercostal nerve (T2). Although it innervates a variable area of skin of the axilla and proximal (medial) arm, it is not part of the brachial plexus and is not covered by a brachial plexus block. The axillary artery lies anterior to the conjoint tendon (which forms the posterior wall of the axilla).

34. **Regarding the orbit:**
    The inferior orbital fissure transmits the zygomatic branch of the maxillary nerve [T]
    The inferior orbital fissure transmits the inferior division of CN 3 [F]
    The supraorbital nerve passes through the supraorbital notch to supply the frontal belly of the occipitofrontalis [F]
    The infraorbital foramen lies in the zygomatic bone [F]
    The infraorbital nerve supplies skin from the lower eyelid to the chin [F]

The inferior orbital fissure is a cleft between the maxilla and the greater wing of the sphenoid. It provides a route of communication between the orbit, the pterygopalatine fossa (medially) and intratemporal fossa (laterally). The zygomatic branch of the maxillary nerve (CN 5.2) passes through it. The inferior division of CN 3 passes through the superior orbital fissure, within the common tendinous ring (and thence the cone of extraocular muscles). The supraorbital nerve is a branch of the ophthalmic division of CN 5 and supplies skin of the upper eyelid, forehead and scalp (the frontal belly of occipitofrontalis is supplied by the temporal branches of CN 7). The infraorbital canal runs from the orbit, through the maxilla, and opens onto the face at the infraorbital foramen. The infraorbital nerve is a branch of the maxillary division of CN 5 and supplies skin from the lower eyelid to upper lip.

35. **The oesophagus:**
    Is approximately 25 cm long in the adult [T]
    Has no outer serosal covering [T]
    Inclines to the right as it descends in the inferior part of the thorax [F]
    Lymph travels relatively large distances in the wall of the oesophagus before reaching the regional lymph nodes [T]
    Drains largely to the systemic venous circulation [T]

As the oesophagus descends through the posterior mediastinum, it inclines to the left below T7 and comes to lie anterior to the descending thoracic aorta before passing through the diaphragm. The (short) abdominal oesophagus drains to the portal circulation: hence an anastomosis exists between the systemic and portal circulation in the lower oesophagus. Chronic portal hypertension can therefore lead to the development of oesophageal varices.

36. **The radial nerve:**
    Is derived from roots C5–T1 [T]
    Provides the principal motor supply to biceps brachii [F]
    Courses around the surgical neck of the humerus [F]
    Gives motor innervation to the medial and lateral heads of triceps brachii [T]
    Can be reliably blocked using ultrasound at the midforearm level [F]

The radial nerve lies in the spiral groove of the humerus (the axillary nerve lies on the surgical neck).

37. **Regarding CN 5 (the trigeminal nerve):**
    It is the largest calibre cranial nerve [T]
    The ophthalmic division provides motor supply to the levator palpebrae superioris muscle [F]

The mandibular division supplies the sensation of taste to the anterior two-thirds of the tongue [F]
Loss of the corneal reflex is consistent with a CN 5 lesion [T]
The mandibular division provides sensory supply to the temporomandibular joint [T]

CN 5 is the largest cranial nerve by diameter and CN 10 is the longest. Levator palpebrae superioris receives motor innervation from the superior division of CN 3 (both somatic and hitch-hiking sympathetic fibres). The mandibular division of CN 5 provides general sensation to the anterior two-thirds of the tongue; the special sense of taste travels with the corda tympani (a branch of CN 7), whose fibres hitch-hike along the lingual nerve (a branch of CN 5.3). CN 5 provides the sensory limb to the corneal reflex, CN 7 the motor limb.

38. Regarding the fetal circulation:
    All of the blood in the umbilical vein enters the right atrium [T]
    The three fetal shunts normally close immediately after birth [F]
    Blood perfusing the brain of the fetus has the same PaO2 as that of the descending aorta [F]
    The foramen ovale remains patent in 25% [T]
    Blood travelling to the fetus via the umbilical vein is fully saturated with oxygen [F]

There are two fetal shunts (not three):

The foramen ovale closes as a result of greater venous return from the lungs to the left atrium, resulting in higher left atrial pressures.

The higher blood oxygen content leads to contraction of the ductus arteriosus, closing the shunt quickly although it takes weeks to months to seal off permanently.

Blood perfusing the fetal brain has a higher PaO2 than that of the descending aorta, which is reduced by the addition of deoxygenated blood from the SVC and right atrium/right ventricle (that has bypassed the lungs via the ductus arteriosus). This mixing occurs distal to the three branches of the aortic arch, from which arise branches supplying the head, neck and upper limbs (brachiocephalic, left common carotid and left subclavian).

39. Regarding the cubital fossa:
    The brachial artery provides the entire blood supply to the hand [T]
    The brachial artery usually divides into the radial and ulnar arteries at the apex of the cubital fossa [T]
    The posterior interosseous nerve arises from the median nerve in the cubital fossa [F]
    Sensory innervation to the medial border of the hand and fifth finger is provided by the median nerve [F]
    The biceps tendon lies medial to the brachial artery [F]

The brachial artery passes through the cubital fossa and divides into radial and ulnar arteries, which give rise to the palmar arches of the hand. The *anterior* interosseous nerve is a branch of the median nerve (the posterior interosseous nerve is a continuation of the deep branch of the radial nerve as it passes between the two heads of supinator muscle). Sensory innervation of the medial border of hand/fifth finger is from the ulnar nerve (which is not found in the cubital fossa). The typical arrangement of structures in the cubital fossa is (from lateral to medial): biceps tendon, brachial artery and then median nerve (TAN).

Section 5: MCQs 1–60 (Answers)

40. **Regarding the nose and paranasal air sinuses:**
    The maxillary air sinus is the largest sinus [T]
    The nasal septum is partly formed from hyaline cartilage [T]
    The blood supply of the septal cartilage is from overlying perichondrium [T]
    CN 1 (olfactory nerve) innervates only the neuroepithelium of the upper nasal cavity (including its roof and upper parts of the medial/lateral walls) [T]
    The nasolacrimal duct drains the lacrimal sac to the inferior meatus of the nasal cavity [T]

Hyaline cartilage has no intrinsic blood supply – nutrients diffuse from capillaries in the overlying perichondrium. Thus, in subperichondral haematoma, blood supply to the underlying cartilage can be compromised and lead to necrosis (resulting in loss of structure, e.g. cauliflower ears when affecting the pinna of the ear).

41. **The following is true of the fetal circulation:**
    50% of the cardiac output passes through the pulmonary capillaries [F]
    Prostaglandin analogues can be used to influence closure of the ductus arteriosus [T]
    The Eustachian valve directs oxygenated blood from the SVC into the pulmonary artery [F]
    The ligamentum teres of the abdomen and the ligamentum venosum are continuous [T]
    The umbilical arteries are obliterated and become the medial umbilical ligament [T]

Although the right ventricle deals with around two-thirds of the cardiac output, only around 10% passes through the pulmonary circulation due to the high resistance and presence of the ductus arteriosus (which shunts blood from the pulmonary artery to the aorta before it reaches the lungs). Prostaglandins can be used to maintain potency of the ductus arteriosus in patients with congenital heart disease (e.g. alprostadil: PGE_1). Prostaglandin antagonists can be used to promote closure (e.g. indomethacin). The Eustachian valve is a fold of endothelium at the junction of the IVC and right atrium, and directs blood entering the right atrium through the foramen ovale and into the left atrium. The ligamentum venosum (intra-abdominal part) and ligamentum teres (part embedded in the posterior surface of the liver) are fibrous remnants of a continuous channel in the fetus. This channel, formed in continuity by the left umbilical vein and ductus venosus, allows oxygenated blood to bypass the liver directly into the IVC. The umbilical arteries extend from the internal iliac arteries to the umbilicus and are thrombosed/obliterated due to high afterload following cord clamping.

42. **The epidural space:**
    Contains the sympathetic chains [F]
    Is continuous with the sacral canal [T]
    Has no lymphatic drainage [F]
    Lies posterior to the posterior longitudinal ligament [T]
    Contains no free fluid in health [T]

43. **Regarding the larynx:**
    The epiglottis is formed from hyaline cartilage [F]
    The superior laryngeal artery pierces the thyrohyoid membrane with the internal branch of the superior laryngeal nerve [T]
    The cricothyroid muscle elongates the vocal cords [T]

The vocalis muscle tenses the vocal cords [T]
The cricoarytenoid joint is a synovial joint [T]

The epiglottis is formed from elastic cartilage, ensuring that it does not calcify and lose its elasticity with age.

44. The lumbar plexus:
Receives a contribution from the L5 nerve root in half of the population [F]
Can be seen as a hyperechoic area within the posterior third of the psoas muscle [T]
Is reliably blocked by the '3 in 1' block [F]
Induces hamstring contraction (knee flexion) as the desired end point/motor response when using a peripheral nerve stimulator to guide correct needle placement [F]
Gives only mixed nerves (with motor and sensory fibres) [F]

The lumbar plexus receives a contribution from T12 in 50% of the population. The desired end point when using a nerve stimulator is the contraction of quadriceps muscle (from stimulation of nerve roots contributing to the femoral nerve). The plexus gives off four mixed nerves and one purely sensory – the lateral femoral cutaneous nerve of thigh (the nerve injured in meralgia paraesthetica).

45. Regarding a sciatic nerve block in the popliteal fossa:
Stimulation of the tibial nerve produces plantar flexion of the ankle/toes and inversion of the foot [T]
Stimulation of the common peroneal (fibular) nerve produces dorsiflexion of the ankle/toes, eversion of the foot [T]
Sciatic nerve block proximally in the thigh will provide anaesthesia and immobility to the knee [F]
The sciatic nerve provides all of the cutaneous innervation to the foot [F]
The posterior cutaneous nerve of the thigh, which provides cutaneous innervation over the posterior thigh and popliteal fossa, is a branch of the sciatic nerve [F]

Knee extension is performed by quadriceps femoris (femoral nerve) and sensation to knee is derived from the femoral (saphenous), obturator and sciatic nerves. The saphenous nerve, a branch of femoral nerve, supplies the medial aspect of foot to the first MTPJ. The posterior cutaneous nerve of the thigh is a branch of the sacral plexus.

46. Muscles whose motor supply is from CN 5 (the trigeminal nerve) include:
Temporalis [T]
Buccinator [F]
Medial and lateral pterygoids [T]
Levator palati [F]
Posterior belly of digastric muscle [F]

Levator palati receives motor supply from CN 10 via the pharyngeal plexus. Only the anterior belly of digastric muscle is supplied by CN 5; the posterior belly is supplied by CN 7.

N.B. Muscles supplied by CN 5:
- Four muscles of mastication: temporalis, masseter, medial and lateral pterygoids

- And four more: two tensors (tensor tympani and tensor palati) and two others (mylohyoid and anterior belly of digastric)

47. **The following is true of the heart:**
    The pericardium is composed of three layers [T]
    In a healthy patient, around 50% of the heart lies to the right of the midline [F]
    The primary chamber comprising the base (posterior surface) of the heart receives four pulmonary veins [T]
    Only 50% of the coronary circulation drains into the coronary sinus [F]
    The coronary sinus contains no valves, thus cardioplegia solution can be injected retrogradely through it to arrest the myocardium [T]

The three layers of pericardium are the fibrous pericardium, and the parietal and visceral layers of the serous pericardium. In health, around one-third of the heart lies to the right of the midline and two-thirds to the left (as illustrated by the surface markings*).

*Surface markings of the heart:
- 3rd right costal cartilage
- 6th right costal cartilage
- 2nd left costal cartilage
- 5th left intercostal space in the midclavicular line

Eighty to ninety per cent of the coronary circulation drains into the coronary sinus; being valveless, retrograde infusion of cardioplegia solution is possible. The so-called 'valve of the coronary sinus' (Thebesian valve), which lies at the opening of the coronary sinus into the right atrium, may prevent some reflux of blood, but is not a 'true valve' as applied to those of the limb veins. The junction of the great cardiac vein and coronary sinus (at the entrance of the oblique vein of Marshall) may be marked by the 'valve of Vieussens'. Again, this is not a true valve and, although it may prevent the passage of catheters down the coronary sinus, it does not appear to obstruct the flow of cardioplegia solution. The Thebesian and Vieussens valves are not always present.

48. **Regarding the structures of the proximal anterior thigh:**
    The femoral nerve is found at the midinguinal point as it enters the thigh, immediately below the inguinal ligament [F]
    The femoral artery is found at the midinguinal point as it enters the thigh, immediately below the inguinal ligament [T]
    The femoral nerve does not supply any structures in the abdominopelvic cavity [F]
    The superficial (anterior) group of femoral nerve branches are purely sensory [F]
    The deep (posterior) group of femoral nerve branches are purely motor [F]

The femoral nerve is located at the *midpoint of the inguinal ligament* (MPIL), which is midway between the ASIS and the pubic tubercle. The femoral artery is located at the *midinguinal point* (MIP), midway between the ASIS and pubic symphysis (the femoral artery therefore lies medial to the femoral nerve). The femoral nerve supplies the iliacus muscle, which arises in the iliac fossa (of the abdominopelvic cavity).

In relation to the femoral nerve branches:
The superficial (anterior) group of the femoral nerve branches comprises two motor and two sensory branches:

- Nerve to sartorius
- Nerve to pectineus
- Medial cutaneous nerve of the thigh
- Intermediate cutaneous nerve of the thigh

The deep (posterior) group of the femoral nerve branches comprises four motor and one sensory branch:

- Nerve to rectus femoris (also supplies hip)
- Nerve to vastus medialis (also supplies knee)
- Nerve to vastus lateralis (also supplies knee)
- Two/three branches to vastus intermedius (one of these goes on to supply articularis genu and knee joint)
- The saphenous nerve (sensory to medial calf and foot as far as the first MTPJ)

49. The internal jugular vein:
Exits the middle cranial fossa through the jugular foramen [F]
The superior, middle and inferior thyroid veins all drain to the IJV [F]
Lies within the carotid sheath [T]
Lies deep to the investing fascia of the neck [T]
Continues as the subclavian vein behind the medial end of the clavicle [F]

The IJV leaves the *posterior* cranial fossa via the jugular foramen. The superior and middle thyroid veins drain to the IJV; but the inferior thyroid vein drains to the brachiocephalic vein. Other tributaries of the IJV include the inferior petrosal sinus (its highest tributary), the pterygoid and pharyngeal plexuses, and the common facial and lingual veins. The IJV joins the subclavian vein to form the brachiocephalic vein behind the medial end of the clavicle.

50. Regarding neurocardiology:
Parasympathetic supply to the heart is only partly from CN 10 (vagus nerve) [F]
The sympathetic outflow to the heart is from spinal levels T1–4 [T]
The autonomic plexus supplying the heart is divided into two parts [T]
The sinoatrial node lies in the wall of the right atrium, just below the SVC [T]
The atrioventricular node lies in the interventricular septum [F]

The parasympathetic nerve supply to the heart is entirely vagal, via the deep and superficial parts of the cardiac plexus. The SA node lies in the wall of the right atrium, just below the SVC and at the top of the crista terminalis. The AV node lies in the interatrial septum, just above the attachment of the septal cusp of the tricuspid valve and to the left of the opening of the coronary sinus.

51. The following are cutaneous branches of the femoral nerve:
Medial cutaneous nerve of the thigh [T]
Intermediate cutaneous nerve of the thigh [T]
Lateral cutaneous nerve of the thigh [F]
Posterior cutaneous nerve of the thigh [F]
Saphenous nerve [T]

Summary of branches and their distribution:
Medial cutaneous nerve of the thigh (L2/3): supplies anteromedial thigh

Section 5: MCQs 1–60 (Answers)

Intermediate cutaneous nerve of the thigh (L2/3): supplies anterior thigh

Lateral cutaneous nerve of the thigh (L2/3): a branch of the lumbar plexus, supplies skin over the lateral thigh

Posterior cutaneous nerve of the thigh (S2/3): a branch of the sacral plexus, supplies skin of the posterior thigh and the leg (to half way down the calf), the lower gluteal region and upper/medial thigh and perineum (via the perineal branch)

Saphenous nerve (L3/4): supplies the anteromedial leg from the knee to the medial malleolus, and the medial side of the foot as far as the first MTPJ

52. **Regarding the dura and venous circulation of the cranium:**
    The tentorium cerebelli lies between the occipital lobes and the cerebellum [T]
    The tentorium cerebelli contains no dural venous sinus in its lateral/posterior (fixed) margin [F]
    The superior petrosal sinus drains the cavernous sinus to the transverse sinus [T]
    Arachnoid villi are protrusions of the arachnoid mater into the subarachnoid space to allow filtration of blood for the production of CSF [F]
    Venous blood from deep regions of the brain drain via the great cerebral vein (of Galen) to the straight sinus [T]

The tentorium cerebelli contains the transverse sinus in its lateral/posterior fixed margin. The superior (fixed) margin of the falx cerebri contains the superior sagittal sinus and the inferior (free) margin contains the inferior sagittal sinus. The inferior petrosal sinus drains the cavernous sinus into the proximal end of the IJV (just below the point at which the sigmoid sinus becomes the IJV). The arachnoid villi protrude through the dura, into the venous blood of the dural sinuses, to allow return of the CSF into the blood. Superficial regions of the brain drain directly to the dural venous sinuses.

53. **Regarding the blood supply of the liver and bowel:**
    The common hepatic artery only supplies the liver [F]
    The superior mesenteric vein drains the foregut [F]
    The midgut extends from the midpoint of the second part of the duodenum to the junction of the proximal two-thirds and distal third of the transverse colon [T]
    The hindgut extends from the distal third of the transverse colon to the upper half of the anal canal [T]
    The portal vein drains deoxygenated blood from the liver to the inferior vena cava [F]

The liver is supplied by the hepatic artery proper: the common hepatic artery is a branch of the coeliac trunk (from the aorta at T12), which gives rise to the hepatic artery proper, the gastroduodenal artery and the right gastric artery. The superior mesenteric vein drains the midgut; the inferior mesenteric vein drains the hindgut. The foregut extends from the mouth to the second part of the duodenum (at the entrance of the ampulla of Vater). The hepatic portal vein drains nutrient rich (but deoxygenated) blood from the gastrointestinal tract (midgut/hindgut) to the liver. The liver then drains to the inferior vena cava via the hepatic veins (right, left and central).

54. **Regarding the popliteal fossa:**
    The short saphenous vein is found in the popliteal fossa [T]
    The sciatic nerve rarely divides proximal to the apex of the popliteal fossa [F]

The sural nerve receives contributions from both tibial and common peroneal (fibular) nerves [T]
The sural nerve runs with the short saphenous vein [T]
Popliteus muscle is supplied by the common peroneal (fibular) nerve [F]

The short saphenous vein enters the popliteal fossa to drain into the popliteal vein. The division of the sciatic nerve is highly variable: although it usually occurs at the apex of the popliteal fossa, the bifurcation may occur anywhere from the gluteal region to within the popliteal fossa. The sural nerve is a branch of the tibial nerve and receives a communicating branch from the common peroneal (fibular) nerve. Popliteus muscle is supplied by the tibial nerve, as are all the muscles of the posterior compartment of the leg.

55. Regarding CN 10 (the vagus nerve):
The left vagus nerve passes over the arch of the aorta [T]
The right recurrent laryngeal nerve enters the thorax before passing under the subclavian artery [F]
The left vagus nerve is a direct relation of the trachea in the thorax [F]
The right vagus nerve contributes predominantly to the anterior vagal trunk [F]
The vagal trunks pass through the diaphragm with the oesophagus at the level of T10 [T]

The right RLN passes under the subclavian artery in the neck (at the thoracic inlet), and it never actually reaches the thorax (unlike the left RLN, which passes under the arch of the aorta in the thorax). The *right* CN 10 is a direct relation of the trachea in the thorax and the *left* CN 10 contributes predominantly to the anterior vagal trunk (the right CN 10 to the posterior trunk).

56. The following is true of spinal nerves:
There are seven pairs of cervical spinal nerves (corresponding to the seven cervical vertebrae) [F]
The dorsal root ganglion contains cell bodies of sensory nerves, but no synapses [T]
The anterior root of every spinal nerve contains both motor and autonomic fibres [F]
A white ramus communicans is associated with every spinal nerve [F]
Both the anterior and posterior divisions (rami) of spinal nerves contribute to the main cervical, brachial, lumbar and sacral plexuses [F]

There are eight cervical spinal nerves (but seven cervical vertebrae). The DRG contains the cell bodies of the first order sensory neurones (pseudounipolar). Sympathetic outflow (thoracolumbar, via white rami communicantes) is from spinal cord segments T1–L2, whereas parasympathetic outflow (craniosacral) is from cranial nerves 3, 7, 9 and 10, plus spinal cord segments S2–4. Therefore, only T1–L2 spinal nerves have a *white* ramus communicans, which carries preganglionic nerve fibres from the spinal cord to the sympathetic chain (paravertebral) ganglia. The great somatic nerve plexuses are derived from the anterior rami of spinal nerves.

57. Regarding innervation of the upper limb:
The ulnar nerve provides motor supply to adductor pollicis [T]
The deep branch of the radial nerve provides sensory supply to the dorsum of the hand [F]

The ulnar nerve provides sensation to the medial aspect of the forearm, proximal to the wrist [F]
Radial nerve palsy, due to fracture of the shaft of the humerus, leads to an inability to extend the elbow joint [F]
The musculocutaneous nerve provides no sensory innervation to the hand [T]

Ulnar nerve innervation of adductor pollicis is the basis for assessing neuromuscular blockade in the upper limb. The deep branch of the radial nerve (the posterior interosseous nerve) provides motor supply to muscles of the posterior compartment of the forearm and is sensory to ligaments/joints only. The superficial branch of the radial nerve provides sensory supply to the dorsum of the hand along with the median and ulnar nerves. There is significant overlap of these territories; the most reliable area for assessing the cutaneous supply of the radial nerve in the hand is over the dorsal aspect of the first web space (an area of skin about the size of a 50 pence piece). The ulnar nerve also provides sensory innervation distal to the wrist: over the palmar/dorsal surfaces of the medial one and a half digits. Motor branches of the radial nerve to the triceps muscles are given off proximally in the axilla, before the radial nerve comes into contact with the shaft of the humerus, so elbow extension may be preserved even if the main trunk of the radial nerve is injured in a fracture of the shaft of the humerus. The musculocutaneous nerve provides sensation to the lateral forearm, via its continuation as the lateral cutaneous nerve of the forearm.

58. CN 12 (the hypoglossal nerve):
    Is a paired nerve comprising both spinal and cranial roots [F]
    Exits the skull through the hypoglossal canal in the temporal bone [F]
    A unilateral lesion of this nerve will cause the tongue to deviate to the unaffected side [F]
    Carries motor and sensory fibres [F]
    Courses through the carotid sheath [T]

CN 12 arises as a series of rootlets from the hypoglossal nucleus in the brainstem. *CN 11 (accessory)* has spinal (cervical) and cranial roots. CN 12 does travel through the hypoglossal canal, though this is situated in the *occipital* bone. A unilateral lesion will cause the tongue to deviate to the *affected* side, which cannot protrude as far due to weakness. CN 12 is entirely motor.

59. Regarding the thoracic spinal nerves:
    The anterior division (ramus) lies anterior to the internal thoracic artery in the upper six intercostal spaces [T]
    The intercostal nerve is the most inferior structure of the main intercostal neurovascular bundle [T]
    They provide a recurrent nerve to the vertebral canal, which provides sensory supply to the dura and arachnoid [T]
    The first intercostal nerve (T1) provides nerve fibres for the brachial plexus but not the first intercostal space [F]
    The second intercostal nerve (T2) provides supply to the axilla [T]

The intercostal nerves lie in a plane external (peripheral) to the arteries, and therefore initially lie posterior to the artery at the back of the space and anterior to it/the internal thoracic artery at the front. In the costal groove, the vein lies above, artery in the middle and nerve below (*remember: VAN*). The recurrent branch also supplies ligaments of the vertebral canal, intervertebral discs, facet joints and vertebral periosteum. T1 provides a main trunk passing over the first rib to the brachial plexus and a branch to the first intercostal space (first intercostal nerve), whilst the lateral cutaneous branch of T2 (intercostobrachial nerve) supplies skin of the axilla.

60. Regarding innervation of the upper limb:
    Sensory innervation to the thumb is provided by the median and radial nerves [T]
    The ulnar nerve supplies skin proximal to the wrist [F]
    The radial nerve supplies all three heads of triceps brachii [T]
    The radial nerve supplies the adductor pollicis muscle [F]
    The median nerve provides the sole motor supply to flexor digitorum profundus [F]

The median nerve provides sensation to the palmar aspect of the thumb and nailbed, with the radial nerve supplying the dorsum. The cutaneous distribution of the ulnar nerve is limited to the hand (i.e. distal to the wrist). The ulnar nerve supplies adductor pollicis (as tested with a peripheral nerve stimulator). Flexor digitorum profundus is supplied by both median and ulnar nerves*.

*The four bellies of flexor digitorum profundus (one continuing as a tendon to each finger) are usually supplied in a 2:2 ratio (median to digits two and three, ulnar to digits three and four). However, this is variable, and the contribution may be 3:1 or 1:3)

References and Further Reading

Multiple previous Royal College of Anaesthetists SAQ exam papers, *British Journal of Anaesthesia Education* articles (formerly *Continuing Education in Anaesthesia, Critical Care and Pain Medicine*) and Anaesthesia Tutorial of the Week editorials were read during the authors' own revision and in the preparation of this book.

The main books reviewed were:

Barker JM, Mills SJ, Maguire SL. *The Clinical Anaesthesia Viva Book*. Cambridge University Press (2009).

Bricker S. *Short Answer Questions in Anaesthesia*, 2nd Edition. Cambridge University Press (2009).

Bricker S. *The Anaesthesia Science Viva Book*, 2nd Edition. Cambridge University Press (2009).

Ellis H, Mahedevan V. *Clinical Anatomy: Applied Anatomy for Students and Junior Doctors*, 12th Edition. Wiley Blackwell (2010).

Ellis H, Lawson A. *Anatomy for Anaesthetists*, 9th Edition. John Wiley & Sons (2014).

Mendonca C, Hillerman C, James J et al. *The Structured Oral Examination in Clinical Anaesthesia: Practice Examination Papers*. TFM Publishing (2009).

Shorthouse J, Barker G, Waldmann C. *SAQs for the Final FRCA*. Oxford Specialty Training (2001).

Sinnatamby C. *Last's Anatomy: Regional and Applied*, 12th Edition. Churchill Livingstone (2011).

Smith T, Pinnock C, Lin T. *Fundamentals of Anaesthesia*, 3rd Edition. Cambridge University Press (2009).

Tandon R. *Structured Oral Examination Practice for the Final FRCA*. Oxford University Press (2011).

Townsley P, Bedforth N, Nicholls B. *A Pocket Guide to Ultrasound-Guided Regional Anaesthesia*. RA-UK (2014).

Index

abdominal wall *see* anterior abdominal wall; anterolateral abdominal wall
achalasia 29, 154
Achilles tendon 70
acromegaly 3, 61
acute myocardial infarction 83
adenocarcinoma 29, 154
Allen's test 5, 74
anaesthesia; *see also* blocks
　acromegaly 61
　carotid endarterectomy 110–111
　eye surgery 144
　inguinal hernia repair 89
　intercostal space 53–55
　larynx 91
　oesophagus 59
　upper limbs 116
　vagus nerve effects 80
anastomoses 153
aneurysms, intracranial vascular 6
ankle
　block 4, 69–70
　nerves 4, 24, 69–70, 145
　structure 70
ansa cervicalis 16, 154–155
anterior abdominal wall 13–14, 101–103
anterior cranial fossa 150
anterior spinal artery syndrome 28, 152
anterior tibial artery 140
anterior triangle, neck 24, 145
anterolateral abdominal wall 16, 24, 112–113, 145
　nerves 113
arcuate ligaments 155
arms *see* upper limbs
arteries
　AV nodal 82
　axillary 149–150
　brachial 157
　carotid 2, 51–52, 77
　common interosseous 149–150
　coronary 81–83

femoral 139–140, 147
hepatic 162–163
lower limbs 139–141
oesophagus 58–59
palmar arches 74
peroneal 147
popliteal 147
radial 74, 149–150
SA nodal 82
spinal 119
subclavian 149–150
tibial 147
ulnar 74
upper limbs 149–150
aspiration 1–2, 44–45
atrioventricular (AV) nodal artery 82
auditory meatus/canal 25, 146–147
auriculotemporal nerve 134
autonomic dysreflexia 25, 146
axillary artery 149–150
axillary block 1, 30, 41–42, 155–156
axillary nerve 116

biceps tendon 157
birth, physiological changes 137
blocks, nerve
　ankle 4, 69–70
　axillary 1, 30, 41–42, 155–156
　brachial plexus 1, 30, 42, 75–76, 155
　caudal 130–132
　epidural 2
　eye 23, 144
　fascia iliaca 2, 49–50
　forearm 100
　interpleural 19, 126
　interscalene 17, 116
　lumbar plexus 3, 56–57
　neuroaxial 29, 131, 154
　paravertebral 12, 97–98
　popliteal fossa 3, 64–65
　rectus sheath 13–14, 101–103
　retrobulbar 144

scalp 20–21, 26, 133–135, 147–148
sciatic nerve 32, 159
sub-Tenon's 144
transversus abdominis plane 16, 113–114, 145
ulnar nerve 13, 100
blood supply
　bowel 33, 162–163
　hand 5, 73–74
　liver 33, 162–163
　lower limbs 22–23, 25, 139–141, 147
　spinal cord 119
　upper limbs 5, 27, 73–74, 149–150
Boerhaave's syndrome 29, 154
bowel, blood supply 33, 162–163
brachial artery 157
brachial plexus 1, 6, 13, 17, 28, 116, 151
　blocks 1, 30, 41–42, 75–76, 153
brain herniation 1, 38
brainstem death organ donation 1, 38–39
breathing/ventilation 14, 105–106
bronchial circulation 26, 149
bronchial tree 1–2, 43–44
bronchial vein 149
Brown–Séquard syndrome 26, 148–149

cardiac structure 8, 32, 81–83, 153–160
carina 24, 44, 148
carotid artery 2, 51–52, 77
carotid endarterectomy 16, 109–111
carotid sheath 28, 152
caudal block 130
　complications and contraindications 131–132
cavernous sinus 86–87
central cord syndrome 27, 150
central tendon 85
cerebellar herniation 1, 38
cerebral artery 6, 77

167

Index

cervical plexus 16, 29, 109–110, 154–155
cervical spine fractures 108
cervical vertebrae 15
chest drains 2, 53–55
circle of Willis 6, 77–78
circulation, coronary 8, 28–29, 81–83, 153–160; *see also* fetal circulation
clavicle 1
common interosseous artery 149–150
coronary arterial dominance 82
coronary artery 81–83
coronary circulation 8, 28–29, 32, 81–83, 153–160
costal cartilages 25, 146, 153–160
costodiaphragmatic/costomediastinal recesses 125
cranium; *see also* skull
  dural venous circulation 33, 162
  fossae 72
  nerves 4–5, 71, 134
  structure 4–5, 72
  sutures 27, 150–151
  trauma 72
cricoid cartilage 145
cubital fossa 19, 31, 127–128, 157
  inadvertent intra-arterial injection 128–129
  superficial veins 128
Cushing's reflex 38

deep cervical plexus 16, 29, 109–110, 154–155
deep peroneal/fibular nerve 70
desmopressin 38–39
diaphragm 8, 29–30, 84–85, 155
dorsal pedis artery 70
dorsal root ganglion 163–164
dural venous sinuses 2, 9, 33, 86–87, 162

endothoracic fascia 150
eparterial bronchus 151
epidural 2
epidural space 2, 31, 46–47, 158
epiglottis 158–159
ethmoid air sinuses 150
ethmoid bone 151–152
extensor retinaculum 70

eye; *see also* orbit
  blocks 23, 144
  muscles 29, 153–154
  nerve supply 23, 144

fascia iliaca, block 2, 49–50
femoral artery 139–140, 147
femoral nerve 33, 56–57, 160–162
femoral triangle 2, 33, 48–49, 161–162
fetal circulation 21, 30–31, 137, 157–158
  changes at birth 137
  foramen ovale 137–138
  paradoxical embolus 138
fetal shunts 157–158
first rib 105
fontanelle 150–151
foramen magnum 1, 37, 46–47
foramen ovale 137–138, 157
frontal bone 151–152

genitofemoral nerve 56–57
great auricular nerve 110, 134
greater occipital nerve 134
groin 2, 33, 48–49, 161–162

hand, blood supply 5, 73–74
heart; *see also* coronary circulation; myocardial infarction
  neurocardiology 33, 161
  structure 8, 32, 81–83, 153–160
hemidiaphragm, raised 85
hepatic artery 162–163
hernia repair, inguinal 10, 20, 89, 130
herniation, brain 1, 38
hypoglossal nerve 34, 164
hypothalamo-hypophyseal portal venous system 3, 61

iliohypogastric nerve 56–57
inguinal region 10, 20, 88–89, 130
innervation *see* nerves
insulin 38–39
intercostal drains 2, 53–55
intercostal space 2, 53–55
intercostobrachial nerve 41–42, 155–156
internal jugular vein (IJV) 2, 32–33, 51–52, 161–162
interpleural block 19, 126

interscalene block 17, 116
  neurological complications 116–117
intra-arterial injection, inadvertent 128–129
intracranial vascular aneurysms 6, 78
intraosseous access 141
ischaemia 153
  spinal cord 18, 120

jugular foramen 7, 80
jugular vein *see* internal jugular vein

knee extension 159

lambda 150–151
laparotomy 2, 47
laryngeal nerves 90–91
larynx 10, 24, 31, 90–91, 146, 158–159
lateral cutaneous nerve 56–57
lateral pectoral nerve 116
lesser occipital nerve 110, 134
levator palati 159
liver
  blood supply 33, 162–163
  structure 11, 92
lower limbs
  arteries 141
  blood supply 22–23, 25, 139–141, 147
  nerves 4
lumbar plexus 3, 32, 49–50, 56–57, 159
  block 3, 56–57
lumbar triangle 24, 145
lumbar vertebrae 15
lungs 1–2, 26, 44–45, 148; *see also* bronchial circulation
  right, root 27, 151

maxilla bone 151–152
maxillary air sinus 150
median nerve 41, 100, 157
methylprednisolone 38–39
mid-inguinal point (MIP) 140, 160–161
midpoint of the inguinal ligament (MPIL) 140, 160–161

Index

muscles
  anterolateral abdominal wall 112–113
  eye 29, 153–154
  intercostal space 53–55
  rectus abdominis 25, 101–102, 147
  trigeminal nerve 32, 159
musculocutaneous nerve 1, 41, 116, 164
myocardial infarction, acute 83
myocardium 82

nasal bone 151–152
nasal cavity 12, 95–96
nasal intubation 12, 96
nasal nerves 95–96
neck, anterior triangle 24, 145
nerves; *see also* blocks
  ankle 4, 24, 69–70, 145
  anterolateral abdominal wall 113
  axillary 116
  cranial 4–5, 71, 134
  diaphragm 85
  femoral 33, 56–57, 160–162
  genitofemoral 56–57
  great auricular 110, 134
  greater occipital 134
  hypoglossal 34, 164
  iliohypogastric 56–57
  intercostobrachial 41–42, 155–156
  laryngeal 90–91
  lateral cutaneous 56–57
  lateral pectoral 116
  lesser occipital 110, 134
  median 41, 100, 157
  musculocutaneous 1, 41, 116, 164
  nasal 95–96
  obturator 49–50, 56–57
  occipital 147–148
  oculomotor 29, 153–154
  oesophagus 58–59
  phrenic 8, 85, 154–155
  pleural membranes 126
  popliteal fossa 33, 163
  radial 13, 30, 41, 99, 156, 164
  recurrent laryngeal 163
  saphenous 69, 145, 159
  scalp 133–135
  spinal 2, 34, 54, 163–164
  supraclavicular 110, 116
  sural 70, 145
  thigh 161–162
  thoracic spinal 34, 164–165
  tibial 69–70
  transverse cervical 110
  trigeminal 18, 30, 121–122, 156–157
  ulnar 41, 100, 164
  upper limbs 13, 34–35, 99–100, 164–165
  vagus 7, 10, 34, 79–80, 91, 163
neuroaxial blocks 29, 131, 154
neurocardiology 33, 161
node of Cloquet 48–49
nose, structure 12, 31, 95–96, 158

obturator nerve 49–50, 56–57
occipital nerve 147–148
occlusive strokes 6, 78
oculomotor nerve 29, 153–154
oesophagus 3, 30, 58–59, 156
  arteries 58–59
  nerves 58–59
  pathology 29, 154
  sphincters 28, 152
  veins 58–59
optic canal 143
orbit; *see also* eye
  margin/rim 28, 151–152
  oculomotor nerve 29, 153–154
  relations 27, 150
  structure 23, 30, 143–144, 156
osteo-ligamentous structure 37

palmar arches 74
palsy 38
paradoxical embolus 138
paranasal sinuses 12, 31, 95–96, 158
paravertebral block 12, 97–98
paravertebral space 12, 27, 97–98, 150
parietal pleura 125, 150
peribulbar block 144
pericardium 153–160
peroneal artery 147
pharyngeal plexus 159
phrenic nerve 8, 85, 154–155
pituitary gland 3, 60–62
pleural membranes 19, 26, 125, 148

costodiaphragmatic/costomediastinal recesses 125
  interpleural block 126
  nerves 126
  surface markings 125
pleuroperitoneal membranes 155
pneumonitis 1–2, 45
popliteal artery 147
popliteal fossa 3, 32, 64–65, 159
  nerves 33, 163
  veins 33, 163
portosystemic anastomosis 11, 92–94
posterior tibial artery 140
proximal anterior thigh 32, 160–161
psoas major muscle 56
pterion 26, 149, 151
pulmonary ligament 148
pulmonary plexus 151

radial artery 74, 149–150
radial nerve 13, 30, 41, 99, 156, 164
raised hemidiaphragm 8
rectus abdominis muscle 25, 101–102, 147
rectus sheath block 13–14, 101–103
recurrent laryngeal nerve (RLN) 163
respiratory tree 1–2, 44
retrobulbar block 144
ribs 14, 25, 104–105, 146
right coronary artery (RCA) occlusion 82
right lung root 27, 151

SA (sinoatrial) nodal artery 82
sacral hiatus 46–47, 131
sacral plexus 159
sacrum 20, 130–131
saphenous nerve 69, 145, 159
saphenous vein 70, 140–141, 145
scalp 20–21
  block 20–21, 26, 133–135, 147–148
  nerves 133–135
sciatic nerve 3, 64
  block 32, 159
secondary cartilaginous joints 108
septum transversum 155
shoulder joints 17

Index

shunts 149
  fetal 157–158
sinoatrial (SA) nodal artery 82
sinuses 150
  cavernous 86–87
  dural venous 2, 9, 33, 86–87, 162
  paranasal 12, 31, 95–96, 158
skull 1, 4–5; *see also* cranium
skull, base 71
sphenoid air sinus 150
spinal artery 119
spinal column 15, 108; *see also* vertebrae
spinal cord 18
  anterior spinal artery syndrome 28, 152
  autonomic dysreflexia 25, 146
  blood supply 119
  Brown–Séquard syndrome 148–149
  central cord syndrome 27, 150
  children 154
  ischaemia 120
  tracts, ascending and descending 119
spinal nerves 2, 34, 54, 163–164
  thoracic 34, 164–165
strokes, occlusive 6, 78
subclavian artery 149–150
sub-Tenon's block 144
superficial cervical plexus *see* cervical plexus
superficial peroneal/fibular nerve 70
superior costotransverse ligament 150
superior orbital fissure 143–144
supraclavicular nerve 110, 116
supraorbital nerve 133
supratrochlear nerve 133

sural nerve 70, 145
sutures, cranium 27, 150–151
synovial joints 108

TAP *see* transversus abdominis plane blocks
tentorium cerebelli 162
Thebesian valve 153–160
thiopentone, inadvertent intra-arterial injection 128–129
thoracic spinal nerves 34, 164–165
thoracic vertebrae 15
thorax 67
thyroid hormone 38–39
tibial artery 147
tibial nerve 69–70
TIPSS *see* transjugular intrahepatic portosystemic shunt
tonsillar herniation 1, 38
trachea 3, 24, 66–67, 146
tracheostomy 3, 67
transjugular intrahepatic portosystemic shunt (TIPSS) 11, 94
transsphenoidal approach, pituitary gland 61–62
transversus abdominis plane (TAP) block 16, 113–114, 145
transverse cervical nerve 110
trefoil tendon 85
trigeminal nerve 18, 30, 121–122, 156–157
  muscles 32, 159
  sensory supply 122
trigeminal neuralgia 122
  causes 123
  management 123

  risk factors, diagnosis 122–123
Tuohy needle 2, 47

ulnar artery 74
ulnar nerve 41, 100, 164
  block 13, 100
umbilical artery 158
umbilical vein 21, 137
upper limbs 13, 17, 99–100, 116
  arteries 149–150
  blocks 13, 17, 99–100, 116
  blood supply 5, 27, 73–74, 149–150
  nerves 13, 34–35, 99–100, 164–165
upper respiratory tract 24

vagus nerve 7, 34, 79–80, 163
  larynx 10, 91
valve of Vieussens 153–160
vasopressin 38–39
veins
  bronchial 149
  cubital fossa 128
  internal jugular 2, 32–33, 51–52, 161–162
  oesophagus 58–59
  popliteal fossa 33, 163
  saphenous 70, 140–141, 145
  spinal 119
  umbilical 21, 137
ventilation/breathing 14, 105–106
vertebrae 15, 108; *see also* spinal column
vestibular ganglion 146–147
visceral pleura 125

Willis, circle of 6, 77–78

zygomatic bone 151–152
zygomaticotemporal nerve 133–134